Vernon Coleman trained as a doctor and practised as a GP for ten years. Now a full time author he has written over twenty books which have been translated into many languages and sold all round the world. He broadcasts frequently on both TV and radio and writes regularly for a number of major newspapers and magazines.

LIFE WITHOUT TRANQUILLISERS

Vernon Coleman

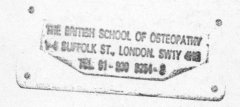

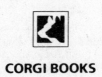

CORGI BOOKS

Dedicated to Anne McDermid and Imogen Parker
with love and thanks

LIFE WITHOUT TRANQUILLISERS

A CORGI BOOK 0 552 12718 3

Originally published in Great Britain by
Judy Piatkus (Publishers) Limited

PRINTING HISTORY
Judy Piatkus edition published 1985
Corgi edition published 1986

This book is set in 10/11pt Imprint

Corgi Books are published by Transworld Publishers Ltd.,
Century House, 61–63 Uxbridge Road, Ealing, London W5 5SA,
in Australia by Transworld Publishers (Aust.) Pty. Ltd.,
26 Harley Crescent, Condell Park, NSW 2200, and in New
Zealand by Transworld Publishers (N.Z.) Ltd., Cnr. Moselle
and Waipareira Avenues, Henderson, Auckland.

Printed and bound in Great Britain by
Cox & Wyman Ltd., Reading, Berks.

CONTENTS

WARNING

If you suffer from any specific mental symptom (such as depression or confusion) then you must see your doctor without delay. You should also seek medical advice if you are in in any way concerned about your health.

LIFE WITHOUT
TRANQUILLISERS

INTRODUCTION

The biggest drug-addiction problem in the world doesn't involve heroin, cocaine or marijuana. In fact, it doesn't involve an illegal drug at all. The world's biggest drug-addiction problem is posed by a group of drugs, the benzodiazepines, which are widely prescribed by doctors and taken by countless millions of perfectly ordinary people around the world.

Although they have been available for less than a quarter of a century, benzodiazepines such as Valium, Librium and Mogadon have become among the most popular drugs in the world. They are so common that if you empty handbags and pockets at any gathering where there are more than half a dozen people present, you'll probably find at least one bottle of these pills. They are used to help people get to sleep, to help people cope with anxiety, and to deal with hundreds of physical and mental symptoms so varied that a full list would look like the index to a medical textbook.

Drug-addiction experts claim that getting people off the benzodiazepines is more difficult than getting addicts off heroin. And yet doctors in hospitals and in general practice continue to write out prescriptions for these drugs. Ten years ago I forecast that the benzodiazepines would prove to be addictive. Medical libraries around the world are stuffed with papers describing the hazards associated with these drugs. And yet *still* they are prescribed in enormous quantities.

Statistics for benzodiazepine consumption are staggering. Figures vary from country to country but on average something like one in every ten individuals takes a benzodiazepine. Despite the fact that these drugs are known to work properly only if taken for a very short period of time, there are millions of people around who have been taking one of these drugs for more than a year. There are, indeed, millions who have been taking benzodiazepines

3

for several years. Most of the long-term consumers are women, and most are over the age of forty, but the numbers of people involved are so huge that no category of human being seems exempt. Men, women, children – they all take benzodiazepines.

For several years now pressure-groups have been fighting to help addicted individuals break free from their pharmacological chains. But the fight has been a forlorn one. As fast as one individual breaks free from one of the benzodiazepines another patient somewhere else becomes addicted.

I believe that the main reason for this is that doctors are addicted to prescribing benzodiazepines just as much as patients are hooked on taking them. I don't think that the problem can ever be solved by gentle persuasion or by trying to wean patients off these drugs. I think that the only genuine long-term solution is to be aware of these drugs and to avoid them like the plague. The uses of the benzodiazepines are modest and relatively insignificant. We can do without them. I don't think that the benzodiazepine problem will be solved until patients around the world unite and make it clear that they are not prepared to accept prescriptions for these dangerous products.

In this book I've tried to do several things. First, I've tried to explain precisely why I think the pressure and stresses in our society are so great that many millions of people need help. Second, I've explained in precise detail just why I don't think that the benzodiazepines provide a safe answer. Much of the research information that I've included here has remained hidden in medical journals around the world until now. Third, I've provided very specific information for those individuals already taking benzodiazepines and wanting to stop taking them. Getting off these drugs is not easy. But it can be done. And finally, I've provided a good deal of information on just how I believe that the individuals suffering from stress and anxiety can cope with their fears and problems more effectively and more efficiently.

I hope this book helps to sound the death knell for the benzodiazepines. But I also hope it offers those millions of individuals using benzodiazepines a viable alternative.

Vernon Coleman, London,
September 1984

Chapter 1.

STRESSES AND CONSEQUENCES

- The special stresses of living in the 1980s
- One man's pressure is another man's pleasure
- What affects our response to stress?
    - Guilt
    - Boredom
    - Vanity
    - Frustration
    - Ambition
    - Fear
    - Lust
- Consequences
- Doctors just cannot cope

The special stresses of living in the 1980s

Most of us get enough to eat, have somewhere warm and dry to sleep at night, don't have to worry too much about being eaten by wild animals and have the choice of several TV channels for entertainment. Compared to our ancestors you'd think we had it made. And yet all the evidence shows that we are in the middle of an enormous epidemic of stress-induced disease. Stress is the twentieth-century equivalent of the plague.

Never before in history have there been so many people needing treatment for such stress-induced disorders as high blood pressure, heart disease and stomach ulcers. Asthma, eczema, colitis and migraine are all stress induced. And millions suffer from sleeplessness, anxiety and other mental manifestations of too much stress. The only reason why Valium and the other benzodiazepines have become so popular is that the epidemic of stress-induced disease has become uncontrollable.

Before discussing Valium itself I want to spend a few pages describing just why I think our peculiar modern stresses have resulted in so much physical and mental disease. We *ought* to be contented, comfortable and happy. But in the developed countries we suffer so much from stress disorders that we have made Valium and similar products the biggest selling drugs of all time.

I think that the explanation for all this is remarkably simple. Our bodies were designed a long time ago. And the sad fact is that they are ill-suited for the type of society and environment which we have now created for ourselves.

Our bodies are designed for a world in which we are surrounded by threatening enemies. We are designed for a world in which fighting and running are useful, practical solutions. Our bodies were originally designed to enable us to cope with confrontations with sabre-toothed tigers. If we meet a specific problem of that sort then we respond quite logically; our muscles tighten, our hearts beat faster, our blood pressure goes up, adrenalin surges through our veins and our bodies are, in general, put on alert. We can then fight, run, jump and climb with astonishing agility.

The trouble is, of course, that today our problems are not quite so simple or straightforward. Instead of being faced with a

7

sabre-toothed tiger, a pack of hungry wolves or an angry boar we are far more likely to find ourselves having to face unemployment, big gas bills or officious policemen. None of these modern problems are easily solved. None can be dealt with by a faster heart beat, a higher blood pressure or tense muscles. Those natural physiological responses won't help you cope more effectively.

And yet that is exactly what your body does. Faced with a threat of any kind your body responds in the only way it knows how – it prepares for physical action. We have not yet evolved fast enough to have learnt that such purely physical responses won't help.

The simple truth is that we have changed our world far faster than our bodies have been able to adapt. At no other time in the history of the world has there been such a constant progression of ideas. Never before have fashions, themes and attitudes changed so rapidly, never before have expectations and pressures been so great. Revolutionary changes in agriculture, navigation, medicine, military tactics, industrial methods, design, transport and communications have all transformed our world. But our bodies are much the same as they were 2,000 years ago. It takes thousands of years for the human body to adapt and we've moved far too quickly for our own good. Today our bodies respond to threats in the same way that they would have responded thousands of years ago. But our responses are now sadly inappropriate.

Indeed, it is your body's natural responses which cause the ill effects produced by stress. And the symptoms of stress-induced disease are produced because the problems that cause the responses do not go away but last for hours, days, months and even years.

If you suddenly find yourself faced with bills that you can't pay, that worry is likely to go on for days and days. And all that time your body will be responding in the only way it knows how – by preparing you for physical action. Aware of the fact that you are under some sort of threat your body will automatically raise your blood pressure, increase your muscle tension and so on. All these changes are designed to help you run away from your bill or fight it to the death.

Unfortunately, instead of helping, such responses merely result in the development of ulcers, heart disease and blood-pressure problems.

One man's pressure is another man's pleasure

The many, varied pressures and problems which we have to face today are usually described by the single word 'stress'. It is a word that is often used inaccurately but it does serve to bring together all the pressures and problems which worry us and put us in jeopardy. The odd thing is, however, that there doesn't seem to be any real correlation between the existence of stress and the development of stress-induced disease. Some individuals seem to suffer enormously when under quite modest amounts of stress, while others are able to cope with enormous stresses and strains – indeed they may even seem to thrive on stress.

The reason for this apparent anomaly is that stress itself never causes any problems at all. It is not the existence of stress that causes damage so much as our *response* to that stress. It is not the changes or the pressures that produce the anxiety or the heart disease but the individual's inability to cope with the difficulties and strains produced by those changes.

Each one of us has two fairly fixed stress thresholds. At one end of the stress spectrum we can all cope with only so much activity. At the other end of the spectrum we can only cope with so much inactivity. If you are a person with a low stress threshold for activity then you are likely to respond badly when you are under pressure. If you have a low stress threshold for inactivity then you will respond badly when you haven't got enough to keep you busy. Boredom will be your downfall.

If the range between your two thresholds is narrow then you're particularly likely to suffer from stress. If the range between your two thresholds is wide then you're likely to suffer relatively little from stress. If you have a narrow stress threshold range then you are particularly likely to end up taking Valium – or one of the other similar drugs.

What affects our response to stress?

Over the years I've slowly come to realise that the way in which we respond to stress is influenced by seven individual driving forces. Those forces are: guilt, boredom, vanity, frustration, ambition, fear and lust. It is these individual forces which decide whether a

9

particular stress ends up producing problems or not. It is these forces which decide whether or not specific worries fall inside or outside your stress threshold range. And, ultimately, it is these seven forces which determine whether or not you'll need Valium.

Because these seven driving forces are so important I've described them on the following pages at some length. It is, by the way, important to understand that any external problem is quite likely to involve more than one of these individual driving forces.

Guilt

Guilt is not just what you feel if you accidentally break a plate in someone else's home. Nor is it simply the emotion you endure should you unintentionally hurt someone's feelings. Guilt is much, much more than either of those things. It is one of life's most powerful, most invasive and most dangerous emotions. And although a certain amount of guilt is caused by regret and wrong-doing, most guilty feelings are inspired not by any dreadful crime but by feelings of inadequacy which have often been produced by others. Sometimes those feelings will have been manipulated intentionally. Sometimes they will have resulted from unconscious manipulations.

Consider, for example, parents who want their daughter to spend Christmas at home. They may well say things like 'If you loved us as much . . .' or 'It will be so lonely without . . .' In both cases they are making her feel guilty. Their manipulative behaviour may or may not be deliberate. Either way the end result will be much the same.

Or consider the young girl who is out on a date with her boyfriend. Settled comfortably in the back of his car they are getting to the stage where there is only one way to go. If she is reluctant he'll probably produce lines such as 'If you loved me . . .' and 'I'll be ill if you don't . . .' Once again, guilt is being used as a manipulative force.

From those two examples you can see that guilt is often built on such foundations as love and compassion. And, indeed, the real irony about guilt is that the kinder and more sensitive an individual is, the more likely he or she will be to suffer from guilt. And it is true too that the closer a relationship the greater the guilt will be. It is in our dealings with immediate members of our families, close

10

friends and lovers that much guilt originates.

Sometimes, the things we say to one another are fairly obviously manipulative. So, for example, such phrases as 'We've made a lot of sacrifices for you . . .', 'We wanted you to have chances we didn't have . . .', and 'You're making your mother ill', are pretty crude. Those are the sort of things that parents will say when they want their children to do something. The chances of their then getting their own way will to a large extent depend on the closeness of the relationship they have with their children. The more devoted parents have been, the easier it will be for them to induce a feeling of guilt in their children.

Although personal relationships are a common and powerful cause of guilt it is, however, also important to understand that guilt can often result from social pressure. I don't just mean the sort of pressures which make us feel guilty if we steal or commit murder. Things are much more subtle than that.

Religious leaders have for centuries recognised and taken advantage of the fact that feelings of guilt can be used to subdue self-confidence and assertiveness and to produce an obedient, malleable congregation. Schoolteachers too will claim, not without reason, that they can mould the minds of young children as if they were made of clay. They frequently use guilt as a weapon.

In addition to teachers and priests, however, there are today very many modern guilt-producing forces. Look around you now and you will probably be able to see several dozen messages designed to make you feel guilty. I'm talking about the sort of messages used by advertising copywriters and if you read or listen carefully to just about any piece of advertising material you'll see what I mean.

So, for example, you'll find phrases such as 'Do you love him enough to buy him . . .', 'Don't your children deserve XYZ breakfast cereal?', 'People will shy away from you if you don't use ABC soap.' In all these instances the advertiser is deliberately trying to make you feel guilty about something so that you will spend money on his product.

Then there are the pressures which come from the political activists such as the Women's Liberation Movement. Now, I'm not suggesting for a moment that anyone who is a member of such an organisation will deliberately try to manipulate you but the fact remains that the ideas put forward by those who support the

11

equality of women in the fullest social, economic and political sense do produce a tremendous amount of guilt.

Women suffer because they have to try and satisfy their well-established desires to look after a husband, children and a home while at the same time trying to establish their own identities as people rather than as wives and mothers. The conflicts between these two aims means that a tremendous amount of guilt is produced. The woman who abandons her career for her family will feel guilty because she will be aware that she is failing herself and her sex. The woman who throws herself wholeheartedly into a career will feel guilty about the time she has to spend away from her home.

Not that this particular type of guilt is unique to women. Men suffer too. Some may feel guilty if they treat a woman as an equal because that conflicts with what they were taught as boys. But many also feel guilty if they treat women as nothing more than delicate, vulnerable, feminine creatures in need of support. Even such a simple decision as whether or not to stand up on a bus and offer a woman a seat can become a cleft stick guaranteeing guilt whichever course is followed.

The influence of guilt is as varied and as difficult to judge as the source. There is, however, little doubt that guilt causes a tremendous amount of shame, inadequacy and inferiority, producing a lack of confidence in many and a feeling of failure in others.

Those feelings are, in turn, responsible for much mental and physical illness.

Boredom

When you think about stress you probably think about harassed business executives struggling across airport terminals with expensive hand luggage clutched in clammy palms. Or red-faced, overweight taxi drivers leaning half out of their cabs and screaming colourful abuse at thoughtless pedestrians. Or nervous, perspiring shop assistants struggling to fend off hordes of frantic shoppers as the winter sales begin. Or of desperate white-faced, white-coated doctors working shoulder to shoulder with teams of bustling nurses as they struggle together to keep an accident victim alive.

That's the sort of image the word stress usually inspires.

And yet the truth is that just as too much activity can cause stress, so *too little* activity can cause stress. As I described at the beginning of this chapter the human body is designed for direct physical action. Too much action and worry of the wrong sort can cause stress. And so can too little. So, paradoxically, one of the most powerful of today's basic driving forces is boredom – a hazard which faces four particular groups of people.

First, there are those individuals whose daily work is uninspiring, undemanding and unrewarding. There once was a time when almost any sort of job required some sort of skill. A craftsman would be expected to have agility in his fingers and skill in his hands. A clerk would be expected to have a facility with words or figures.

Today, however, there are many millions of individuals whose work demands nothing more than that they act as nursemaids to pieces of machinery. In offices there are computers and word processors which can write letters, check spelling, add up numbers and keep files. They can do these tasks far more efficiently and far faster than any individual could hope to do them. In factories there are pieces of machinery which can turn out an endless stream of carefully polished, finely balanced objects. No single craftsman working with a lathe and his own skills could hope to emulate such accuracy.

Modern machines are, indeed, so sophisticated that they are invariably the principals in any working relationship. Conveyor belts carry raw materials from one part of the factory floor to another and the whole process of manufacture will be geared to the needs, capabilities and strengths of the machines rather than the men and women operating them. Men who might have once been regarded as skilled craftsmen are employed as simple machine minders. Instead of doing work from which they can derive pride and satisfaction they babysit huge pieces of complicated engineering which have an insatiable appetite for raw materials and electricity but which allow the individuals operating them little opportunity for pride or self-expression.

It is this same race to replace skilled workmen with machines which has led to the second enormous cause of boredom in our society – unemployment. If a company is to compete on an international scale it must install more and more machinery. And

13

that must inevitably lead to growing unemployment.

Because we live in a job-orientated society where a man's status and even masculinity depend on his having a job with some position and some power, unemployment produces a number of damaging forces. The man who has lost his job or who is unable to find a job will undoubtedly feel a tremendous sense of guilt, for example. He will feel that he has failed himself and all those around him. But there will also be boredom. The days are long for a man who has no job.

The third group of individuals who suffer tremendously from boredom include those men and women who have voluntarily retired. For several years now I have regularly read reports of trade-union officials who have been noisily campaigning for earlier retirement for their members. At the same time I have seen a steady stream of men and women in their fifties and sixties shuffling through my surgery complaining bitterly about the fact that they have retired too soon.

What those trade-union officials do not realise is that even when a job is dull and monotonous it still offers something to the man or woman who does it. The simplest, least demanding job of all still offers something in the way of friendship, companionship, authority and meaning. A man may complain about his job, his employer and his working conditions but at least he has something positive to complain about. Too often the man or woman who has retired too soon and without adequate preparations won't have even that.

Finally, I must not leave the problem of boredom without mentioning the housewife. She, perhaps more than any other single group of individuals in our society, is a modern-day victim of this unexpected and underestimated type of pressure. Talk to any doctor about the sort of people who are the most common users of the benzodiazepines and he will almost certainly tell you about the women who are generally (and often rather patronisingly) dismissed as 'mere' housewives. They are often bored out of their minds.

Living in a comfortable house in a pleasant area and seemingly happily married with a healthy family of her own the average housewife may well be bored silly by the relentless and undemanding nature of her life. (In addition, she may well feel

14

guilty about feeling dissatisfied.) It may be difficult to get a job, to get out of the house, to have any sort of stimulating conversation and to feel in any way fulfilled as an individual.

As a stress-producing force boredom is invariably under-estimated. It is, however, one of the most significant of these seven forces.

Vanity

Why did you spend so long in the bathroom this morning? Why did you take care deciding what to wear? Why did you get so upset when your car acquired a small dent on the nearside wing? And why did you buy that bag you couldn't afford when the cheaper one without the designer label looked just as good? Why do you always put fresh underclothes on when you visit the doctor? Why do you get upset if you think people underestimate your intelligence? Why do you get offended if you think someone is only after your body? Why do you feel ashamed of the fact that your command of languages isn't as good as it ought to be? Why do you laugh at jokes that you don't understand? Why do yo insist on nodding wisely when people talk about physicists, painters and musicians you have never heard of?

It's vanity.

Why is a woman upset if she finds herself attending a party where another woman is wearing an identical dress? Why do women spend so much time at the hairdressers? Why do so many women worry about the size and shape of their breasts? Why do many women spend so much money on 'wrinkle-erasing' creams?

It's vanity.

Why do so many men and women spend so much time and effort trying to lose weight and stay slim? Why is there a multi-million-pound industry selling dietary advice, diet foods, magic diet pills and specialist books on the subject.

It's vanity.

Why do men worry when they start to go bald? Why do men worry so much about the size of their penises? Why do men worry if they don't have hair on their chests? Why do men worry about the size of their offices and whether or not their secretaries have carpets on their floors? Why do men always want the key to the executive

15

washroom? Why do men over forty always feel flattered when young girls stop and talk to them?

It's vanity.

So, to a certain extent, of course, vanity is a natural phenomenon. We all feel a certain amount of pride in our appearance, our intelligence, our success and our status.

But vanity isn't entirely natural. For the very simple reason that there are many people who have a vested interest in *encouraging* us to be vain.

So, there are the beauty experts telling us how we should look, the dress designers telling us what we should wear, the plastic surgeons promising eternal youth, the hairdressers offering good looks and many suitors, and the car manufacturers offering admiring glances and envious neighbours. And an endless stream of other professionals all anxious to encourage us in our vanities and ever ready to help us spend our money satisfying our inner needs and repelling our insecurities.

Your vanity is someone else's big business these days.

Frustration

There has been a power cut. You are sitting shivering in your gadget-filled kitchen while you struggle to read a day-old newspaper by the flickering light of a lonely candle stub. You dare not open the fridge in case the power cut is prolonged and the food inside ruined by warmth. The television set does not work. Nor does your wireless or casette player. The washing is half done and the gas central-heating boiler has switched off. You can't get any hot water to make a drink because you have got an electric cooker and a useless electric kettle. Your immersion heater won't work so you can't take a soothing bath.

That is frustration.

You are sitting in a new car watching the driver in front pick his nose and fiddle with his ear lobes. You have been watching him for thirty minutes. The traffic jam of which you are just one small part seems to stretch for miles. There doesn't seem to be any end to it. A cheerful voice on the radio has just informed you that the hold-up is likely to continue for another ninety minutes.

That is frustration.

You are standing at a bus stop in the pouring rain with your arms piled high with paper packages. Four buses go past. They are all headed for somewhere other than your destination.

That is frustration.

You need to make a telephone call urgently. Every call box you enter is either broken or out of order. The only telephones which are working are being used.

That is frustration.

You are looking for a parking space in town. When at last you see one you accelerate with delight in your heart. Then you discover that someone has left a motorcycle parked in the space.

That is frustration.

You are at Athens airport waiting for an aeroplane to Manchester. You've been there for three hours and you don't have any Greek money left. Then there is a public announcement that the plane you are due to catch has been delayed because a plane heading for Turin from Paris has had an engine failure.

That is frustration.

You are trying to sell your house. You think you have finally managed to complete a deal. More important you have discovered a dream house that you want to buy. It's got everything you ever wanted at a price you can afford. The deal is about to go through. Then, at the last moment, the whole carefully constructed chain of exchanges falls apart when the people who are due to buy the house that the people who are buying your house are selling can't get a mortgage.

That is frustration.

It is Christmas morning and someone has brought you an electronic gadget. It is something you have always wanted but never been able to afford. You are really pleased. Then you discover that it hasn't got any batteries in it. And the shops are shut.

That is frustration.

It would be possible to go on and on making a list of similarly frustrating episodes. The truth is that our lives are now so complex, and we are so dependent on one another, that hardly a day goes by without our being severely inconvenienced in one way or another. A temporary breakdown on the other side of the world can cause havoc thousands of miles away. A strike by one group of workers can cause frustrations for thousands or even millions of workers who don't seem to have anything in common with the people involved in the first dispute.

And the more complex our lives become, the more we become dependent on other people, the more sophisticated the equipment upon which we rely, the more catastrophic the frustrations will become.

Ambition

The pressure to achieve starts earlier and earlier. Stand outside a junior school at four in the afternoon and you will see a steady stream of children hurrying out with their briefcases and satchels stuffed to the buckles with text books, exercise books, calculators and homework schedules.

Follow those same children to the sports field on a games afternoon and you will see them being bullied and harried into action. It is no longer enough to compete or play the game. The important thing is to win. And it is vital to have that burning yearning to succeed, to be first, to be the best and to be the star performer.

Shakespeare said that some men are born great, some achieve greatness and some have greatness thrust upon them. Today the same can be said about ambition: some men are born ambitious, some achieve ambition and some have ambition thrust upon them.

Today, success is a watchword that few can dare to despise. Only the truly successful can pretend to ignore the need to fuel their ambition with raw aggression and ruthless determination. If you are born with ambition then your energy and fire will win respect and admiration from others. If you are born without ambition you will be encouraged to achieve it. The social, economic and material advantages of fulfilled ambition will be explained in endless detail. And if you are born without ambition and you fail to achieve it you will still not escape. As the years go by you will have it thrust upon you as you gradually learn that ambition is the only salve for the wounds created by envy, covetousness and simple admiration.

It is ambition that leads the teenage scholar to push himself or herself so hard that a mental breakdown is inevitable. It is ambition that forces parents to thrust a tennis racket into the hands of their six-year-old and stand over him as he practises for four, five or six hours a day. It is ambition that pushes a man or woman to spend twelve hours a day in the office and to then set off for home clutching a briefcase full of papers. It is ambition that inspires a would-be writer to sit down, mentally and physically exhausted after a hard day's work, and to tap at a typewriter on the kitchen table, endeavouring to produce a best-selling novel.

It is ambition that inspires a man to sell his home and his car so that he can gamble the proceeds on a business venture that may cost him everything. It is ambition that encourages an individual to push himself so hard, so relentlessly and so single-mindedly that he burns himself into a stale, lifeless, grey shadow of his former self.

It is ambition that makes you dissatisfied with your reliable four-year-old car, your battered but effective washing machine, your serviceable but threadbare stair-carpet and your happy seaside holidays in a caravan. It is ambition that encourages thousands of women to put up with unwanted passes and sexual harassment from their bosses. It is ambition that pushes men and women into leaving jobs they enjoy and taking jobs they don't want – just because the pay is better and there is more power attached.

It is ambition that turns pleasant, gentle, peaceful people into rude, aggressive, demanding people.

We used to be driven by hunger. That was the dominant emotion in a world where food was in short supply and life was simply a question of survival. Today we have learned to acquire more sophisticated tastes and desires. Encouraged by the advertising copywriters (who are ever anxious to persuade us to buy bigger and better things), by the politicians (always eager to tell us that we can have it better), by the fashionable men and women of the media (endlessly searching for new fashions, new trends and new ideas), we have learned to acquire an insatiable ambition for something better.

It is the very insatiability of our ambition that produces such pressure and such pain. There is no end, no solution, no answer and no cure for our ambition. The search and the drive must go on endlessly.

Fear

Stone Age man was lucky as far as fear was concerned. Sure, he had to worry about the wild animals out for his blood and he had to worry about not getting enough to eat. But there wasn't much else.

19

There may have been occasional problems with other Stone Age men. But none of his problems were too complicated. And none were problems that he couldn't do something about.

Today we have much, much more to be worried about.

Take health for example. There are millions of ways in which you can learn to worry about your health. Listen to the experts arguing about what is good for you – or bad for you – and you will soon start to feel those twinges of fear nibbling at your very soul. Fats are good for you, say some. No, fats are bad for you, say others. You must exercise more. But don't exercise too much. Don't smoke. Don't drink. Don't get bored. Get busy. But don't do too much. Don't drink too much tea or coffee. And don't use sugar at all. Eat plenty of fresh vegetables. And bran. And fruit. But not bananas. Check your own blood pressure regularly. But don't get obsessed with your health. That will be bad for you too. Have X-rays done at least once every six months. But watch out for the radiation. Trust your doctor. But don't take any of the pills he prescribes for you.

If you are feeling ill then visit an acupuncturist. Or a herbalist. Or a homoeopath. Or a naturopath. Or an osteopath. Or a pharmacist. Or your mother. Or your own doctor. Or any doctor. Or an aromatherapist. Or a faith healer. Or a psychotherapist. Or a chiropodist.

Buy a bottle of aspirin tablets. Or an iron tonic. Or vitamin capsules. Or vitamin E ointment. Protein tablets perhaps. Or paracetemol. Or more ginseng. Or cabbage. Or spinach. Or a decongestant.

And so it goes on. Switch on the TV and you'll see an expert telling you what is good for you. And what will kill you. Switch channels and you'll see another expert telling you exactly the opposite. With equal conviction. Switch on the radio and you'll hear someone else making promises and threats that he will never be able to fulfil. Open a magazine and there is more advice. Open a newspaper and there are details of fantastic breakthroughs and horrifying new dangers. It is hardly surprising that we are all becoming certified hypochondriacs, all desperately frightened for our future good health.

Not that our health is the only thing we are encouraged to worry about.

There is inflation.
And the nuclear question.
And the political situation in the Middle East.
And the price of tomatoes.
And the melting polar ice cap.
And the problem of apartheid.
And the price of beef.
And the problem of inner-city violence.
And the price of bread.
And the quality of the ionosphere.
And the polluted seas.
And the political situation in China.
And the price of milk.
And the energy crisis.
And the erosion of the coastline.
And the price of petrol.
And the number of hi-jackings in America.
And the crisis in Poland.
And the rising unemployment figures.
And the amount of violence in the suburbs.
And the price of coffee beans.

Fear is a way of life for most of us. We are encouraged to worry, and to keep us uncertain, apprehensive and nervous, we are supplied with new themes each day.

Lust

Lust is a pretty basic human emotion. Few of our ancestors can claim to have remained immune to the group of simple yearnings collectively classified as lust.

But lust has not remained unaffected by modern influences and it is today a far more sinister and far more powerful emotion than it was when it first won a place in the original seven deadly sins.

Today we are encouraged to follow our primitive instincts by an extraordinarily varied set of forces. There is, for example, the pressure that comes from the many commercial interests with a financial incentive to draw our attention to the feelings of lust which might otherwise have remained unnoticed.

To begin with, of course, there are the more primitive

entrepreneurs who publish, market and sell glossy magazines containing nude photographs of either men, women or both depending upon their intended market, the owners of certain nightclubs, the producers and directors of pornographic films and the purveyors of vibrators, crotchless panties, rubbing oils, transparent black negligees and other titillating items.

The influences of these commercial enterprises are, however, strictly limited. Their sales are relatively small, their turnover unsubstantial and their customers measured in mere single figure millions.

It is the subtler salesmen who are more powerful and more effective. The enormous international industries who use sex to sell their cars, their washing machines, their soap powders, their deodorants, their jeans, their shoes, their perfumes, their hair dyes, their paperback novels, their holiday villas, their daily newspapers, their moisturising creams, their suntan oils, their nail varnishes, their sports jackets, their luggage, their headscarves, their motor bikes, their sailing boats, their cigarettes, their wines, their hard liquors, their soft drinks, their cream buns, their chocolates, their stockings, their shirts, their blouses, their talcum powders, their hotels, their long-playing records, their briefcases, their lipsticks . . .

The advertising slogans are clever, the photographs are tasteful, the models look somehow demure and yet experienced, the locations are exotic, the circumstances erotic and the implications undisguised. Buy this product, the advertisers claim, and your life will be enriched. Live without that product, and you will remain second-rate and life will pass you by.

Together with these promises and threats, however, there are other more important implications. For there is always that underlying assumption that you will be influenced by the sexual hints and notions contained within those advertising slogans. The suggestion is that if you are not constantly thinking about sex and not always prepared to respond to the slightest tremor of promise, then you must be deprived, inadequate or, worse yet, simply unresponsive.

Before the international multi-corporations started using sex to sell their products lust was just another sin. It was no more important to most people than envy or sloth. It was something everyone knew existed, something most people learn to live with, and something allowed out on Saturday nights.

With the lipstick-sportscar-cigarette-soft drink advertising revolution, all that has changed. The advertisers told us that we should be thinking about sex all the time. They insisted that we should be constantly aware of our sexual desires. And they taught us that we should be equally aware of the desires and inclinations of those around us. Most important of all they led us to understand that if we did not spend our waking days trying to work out ways to seduce our neighbours then there must be something sadly wrong with us.

Lust used to be an optional extra.

The international multi-corporations changed all that. And made it a necessity. So, today, many people feel that if they are to behave and think as everyone else behaves and thinks then they must be forever conscious of sex and that if they don't think constantly of rounded buttocks, heaving breasts and bulging groins then they must be sadly inadequate.

Consequences

People don't usually turn up at the doctor's surgery complaining of any of the seven deadly forces, of course. It is not until physical or mental symptoms appear that most people seek help. It would not be possible to make a totally comprehensive list of all the symptoms resulting from stress but I have compiled a short list of some of the commoner problems which result when an individual's stress threshold has been breached.

Physical symptoms include:

allergies	diarrhoea	indigestion
alopecia	digestive	impotence
appetite loss	problems	itching
arthritis	dizziness	menstrual
asthma	duodenal	problems
backache	ulceration	migraine
bed wetting	eczema	nausea
blood pressure	fainting	obesity
colitis	gastritis	palpitations

23

constipation	hay fever	tremors
cough	headaches	ulcers
cystitis	heart disease	vomiting
dermatitis	heartburn	wheezing

Mental symptoms include:

anxiety	irritability	personality
crying	memory failure	disorders
depression	nervous	phobias
fear	breakdown	stuttering
hysteria	nightmares	tension
insomnia	obsessions	

Doctors just cannot cope

Visit a doctor with any of the symptoms mentioned on either of these two lists and there is a very good chance that you will come away with a prescription for Valium or one of the other benzodiazepines.

The reason for this is remarkably simple: doctors just don't know how else to cope.

Before the Second World War most doctors spent most of their time dealing with purely physical problems. They dealt with pains and bleeding, breathlessness and infections, and they treated such straightforward problems as heart disease, pneumonia and fractures. Medical training was designed for this sort of problem.

It wasn't until the 1950s and 1960s that the type of problem being discussed in the doctor's surgery began to change and doctors became aware that stress and anxiety could have a profound influence on the development of apparently simple physical disorders.

The stresses and strains of life in the post-war years had changed the whole face of medicine and suddenly doctors found that they were expected to deal with mental and psychological problems. They found themselves facing patients who were anxious, depressed, irritable, upset and often just miserable. They found themselves being asked to treat problems such as insomnia, baby battering and general nervousness.

Even more important than all this, however, they found themselves being told to look for physical signs of mental distress. Suddenly it became widely known that a whole range of apparently simple physical problems were, in fact, either caused or made worse by stress. And the new medical dilemma was accentuated by several other changes too.

First, there was the fact that in the post-war years families began to move apart. New towns were built, new housing estates sprang up and instead of being able to pop next door for advice, young couples (and in particular young women) found themselves hundreds of miles away from family support. The result was that a growing number of people began to look for professional help and to lean on their doctors far more than they ever had done before.

The second factor that had a tremendous influence on the demand being made of the medical profession was the change in attitude that was encouraging millions of men and women to regard mental problems (and physical problems associated with mental worries) not as something that had to be borne but as something that could be treated. Encouraged and inspired by over-enthusiastic doctors, psychiatrists and psychologists, scores of magazine and newspaper articles appeared in which readers were told that anxiety could be treated, that they did not have to put up with depression, and that the symptoms of mental exhaustion which had in the past been regarded as just part of life could be cured. Millions were encouraged to believe that they need never endure anything remotely resembling unhappiness. Millions honestly believed that they were entitled to an anxiety-free life. The relationship beween stress and disease became common knowledge. And the impact in the surgery was tremendous.

The truth, however, was that doctors were neither prepared for, nor capable of coping with the sudden demand for help with psychiatric problems and stress-related diseases.

They weren't prepared for such demands because most of them had been trained in medical schools where psychiatry was still regarded as something of an oddity and where the amount of time devoted to the study of psychiatric problems was probably less than the amount allocated to the study of rare tropical diseases. Medical schools are always slow to adapt or change their teaching emphasis,

25

and up until very recently psychiatry was regarded as very much a fringe subject.

The other reason why doctors could not cope was horrifyingly simple. Despite the fact that many programmes and articles had given the impression that great advances had been made in the diagnosis and treatment of psychiatric problems with stress-related diseases, the truth was (and indeed still is) that psychiatrists and neurophysiologists still know very little about how the brain works, hardly anything about what happens when things go wrong, and next to nothing about what to do when symptoms of mental illness do exist. If this claim sounds too extreme then I suggest that you flick through any pair of recent psychiatric textbooks or examine a few medical journals published in recent months. You will quickly see that psychiatry is one area of medicine where experts virtually never agree. Some psychiatrists still believe that brain surgery is the answer to many mental problems. Others argue that cutting out bits of brain is like tearing bits out of the TV set when the picture is distorted. Some psychiatrists believe in the value of Electro-Convulsive Therapy. Others claim that the whole practice is barbaric. Some psychiatrists argue that severely ill patients need to be kept locked up. Others say they should be allowed out free in the community.

So, back in the 1950s, doctors suddenly found themselves facing a new epidemic that they couldn't cope with, and found their surgeries filled with patients who probably knew as much as they did about the relationship between stress and illness.

The answer to all their prayers came with the discovery of a new group of drugs called the benzodiazepines.

In the next chapter I'm going to explain just how these drugs first came on to the market.

Chapter 2.

PROSPECTS AND PROMISES – THE ARRIVAL OF VALIUM

- A drug is born
- How do the benzodiazepines work?
- What do the benzodiazepines do?
- How your body deals with them
- The family grows
- The benzodiazepines – a much-needed solution
- Why did doctors accept the benzodiazepines so uncritically?
- Helped by the reaction against the barbiturates
- Just how many benzodiazepines are there altogether?
- Am I taking a benzodiazepine?
- Are the many benzodiazepines different?
- How popular are the benzodiazepines?
- The prescribing explosion still continues
- The benzodiazepines in hospitals
- The benzodiazepines in general practice
- What of the future?

A drug is born

Any major international drug company which wants to acquire and hold a profitably sized chunk of the market for prescription drugs must spend a considerable amount of time and money on research. Multi-million-pound companies cannot just sit around waiting for good ideas to fall out of trees – they all have large, well organised research departments where skilled scientists constantly search for new products. These scientists share one hope; that the drug they are about to discover will be a revolutionary product which will save the world, enrich the company and make their reputation.

Although looking for new drugs is usually a tiresome, unromantic activity, the discovery of an important new product will invariably owe a great deal to chance and good fortune. Although routine must be followed and the research process continued methodically, working scientists know only too well that when a new and remarkable drug is found the story of that product's discovery and development will invariably include more than a touch of imagination, flair and simple good luck.

The story of the discovery of the benzodiazepines is no exception. As described by Professor Irvin M. Cohen in an essay entitled 'The Benzodiazepines', which appeared in *Discoveries in Biological Psychiatry* (published by Lippincott in 1970) it is clear that the Valium story started back in the 1930s when Dr Leo H. Sternbach was working as a research assistant at the University of Krakow in Poland. Dr Sternbach was at the time involved in a theoretical study of the chemistry of benzophenones and heptoxdiazines. These weren't new substances – they had been discovered at the end of the nineteenth century and their structure had been fairly clearly defined in the mid 1920s.

Although the story starts there, in Poland, there was a huge gap before anything of importance happened. After working on these products in the 1930s Dr Sternbach did little more on them until 1954 when, working in America at the New Jersey laboratories of Hoffman La Roche, and inspired by the huge commercial success of such early tranquillisers as the phenothiazine derivatives and meprobomate, he began to look at them again – this time in the hope that they might prove to have some sort of pharmacological action on the brain.

29

The choice of the benzophenones and heptoxdiazines was not mere chance. When studying chemicals in the hope that they will prove to have useful properties, a research chemist usually tries to work with substances which are fairly easy to get hold of, which can be fairly readily changed into new substances and which can be produced in the laboratory in fairly large quantities. The heptoxdiazines fitted the bill perfectly.

After producing some forty new products, however, Dr Sternbach was close to giving up with this particular group of chemicals. None of the substances he had created had any pharmacological action. He was so disillusioned and disappointed by his failure to find anything exciting that the result of his last experiment – which was called Ro5-0690 – was put on a shelf while he turned his attention to other research projects.

There then followed another gap of eighteen months before anything else happened. Then, when the laboratory was being given a spring-clean a chemist working with Dr Sternbach suggested that Ro5-0690 should be properly tested. It was duly sent off to Roche's Director of Pharmacological Research and two months later, in July 1957, a report was produced describing the substance as being a hypnotic, a sedative and a muscle relaxant. By March of 1958 the structure of this new, remarkable and promising compound had been identified as 1,4-benzodiazepine. It was found to be an entirely new chemical substance.

From that point on the new product was the subject of intense investigation.

Excitement grew when it was discovered that this new compound was so powerful that it could tame wild animals. The initial euphoria was then temporarily replaced by some disappointment when it was also shown that when given to elderly patients the drug caused unpleasant side effects. For a while, 1,4-benzodiazepine was nearly dismissed as a fairly ordinary and commercially unpromising sedative.

A couple of months later, however, Roche decided to do some more trials with their new substance. One of the doctors invited to test the new drug was Dr Irvin M. Cohen in Galveston. He quickly found that Ro5-0690 was effective in controlling both tension and anxiety and that it did so with relatively few side effects. The other researchers testing the drug, Dr Titus H.

Harris at the University of Texas Medical Branch in Galveston and Dr James R. Sussex who was then at the University of Alabama School of Medicine in Birmingham, also found that chlordiazepoxide, as the substance had by then been christened, showed distinct promise.

At a meeting at the University of Texas Medical Branch in Galveston in November 1959, the drug's properties as a muscle relaxant, anti-convulsant and treatment for anxiety were described. On February 24 1960 the American Food and Drug Administration approved the drug, on March 12 1960 the first published note describing the drug appeared in the *Journal of the American Medical Associaton,* and later that same month chlordiazepoxide was launched to the medical profession.

It was known as Librium.

How do the benzodiazepines work?

Although the early clinical research work done on chlordiazepoxide showed quite emphatically that the drug had an effect on human patients, when it was first launched no one really knew exactly how chlordiazepoxide worked, nor what effects it had on human beings. The research programme initiated to test the new drug had shown that the benzodiazepines reduced anxiety and muscle tension but had not revealed precisely how this action was achieved.

Since then many books and research papers have been written about the possible activities of the benzodiazepines. We still do not know precisely what happens when the drug is absorbed into the body or what long-term effects it may have, but we do now know a little about some of its actions.

First, for example, we know that the benzodiazepines are well absorbed into the human body. They can be taken by mouth, inserted in suppository form, or given by injection. Their ready solubility in fat means that they can travel around inside the body with considerable ease – getting into the tissues of the brain quite readily.

What happens when they get into the brain is more of a mystery. It has been known for some time that the benzodiazepines change the rhythm of the electrical activity within the brain

31

and it has been recognised that they have a powerful effect on a number of naturally occurring substances. So, for example, when someone takes a benzodiazepine the amount of noradrenaline present in his brain changes. There are effects too on the quantities of dopamine, serotonin and central monoamines present in the brain and it has been suspected for some time that by changing the amount of these substances present the benzodiazepines may affect an indivdiual's mood.

Transmitters which carry messages from one part of the brain to another are affected too and it has been proved that the benzodiazepines have an influence on a substance called gamma-aminobutyric acid which is present in large parts of the human central nervous system and is believed to be a vital link in the system designed to carry messages around the brain. There is evidence too that the benzodiazepines have an effect on glycine neurons which also play a part in the transmission of impulses within the brain.

Of all the evidence which exists about how the benzodiazepines work the most exciting has undoubtedly been that which has shown that there are within the brain special receptors which seem to be formulated in such a way that they can respond only to drugs in the benzodiazepine group. If this research is correct then it is possible that a natural Valium-like substance exists within each one of us.

What do the benzodiazepines do?

Since they were first introduced into clinical practice at the start of the 1960s it has been known that the benzodiazepines have four most important actions.

First, and perhaps most important, they relieve anxiety.

Second, they have a sedative action and make people who take them feel sleepy. Whether they produce sleepiness by decreasing restlessness, irritability and anxiety, or whether they have some specific hypnotic properties of their own, is still something for the research workers to worry about.

Third, some of the benzodiazepines (diazepam in particular) have an anti-convulsant effect and are widely used in the treatment of conditions such as epilepsy. There is still some argument about whether the benzodiazepines produce their anti-convulsant action by some specific action on parts of the brain or simply as a side effect of their sedative, anxiolytic effect.

Finally, the benzodiazepines are known to be able to relax tensed and tight muscles. They have been used in the treatment of various degrees of muscle rigidity – sometimes with great success.

How your body deals with them

Once they have been in the body for a few hours the benzodiazepines, like most drugs, are broken down into other substances. One of the substances most commonly produced in this way is something called desmethyldiazepam – a chemical which is known to continue to act in the body for about 100 hours.

Because the breakdown substances produced when the benzodiazepines are destroyed can survive for so long and can continue to have an effect for such a long period of time the amount of drug in the body can steadily accumulate if benzodiazepines are taken for many days or weeks.

So, for example, if you take one benzodiazepine tablet on a Monday then you'll have just that one benzodiazepine tablet circulating in your blood.

If you then take a second tablet on Tuesday you'll have the breakdown products from Monday's drug to add to your new tablet. You'll have a larger amount of the drug in your blood.

Add another fresh tablet on Wednesday and you'll end up with an even higher blood concentration. You'll have Monday's drug residue, Tuesday's drug residue and Wednesday's fresh drug to affect your body and brain.

And so it goes on. By Friday you'll have left-over products from Monday, Tuesday, Wednesday and Thursday circulating in your body.

The family grows

Even before Librium had hit the drug stores, the prescription pads and the first patients' stomachs, the Roche research laboratories were busily hunting for variations on their promising theme. They knew that if they remained content with their one effective benzodiazepine, other competing drug companies would start experimenting and would be able to manufacture their own versions of this promising drug. It was sound commercial sense for Roche to hurry to discover and patent as many benzodiazepines as possible. Diazepam was one of these.

It was quickly discovered that diazepam wasn't just as good as chlordiazepoxide but that it was in some circumtances even better. So, for example, it was found that it was five times as potent a tranquilliser, that it was five times more effective as a muscle relaxant and ten times stronger as an anti-convulsant. In 1963 Roche launched diazepam as the drug Valium.

Meanwhile another drug company, Wyeth Laboratories, had started investigating the benzodiazepines. Their first drug in this group was oxazepam. Before the end of the 1960s many other manufacturers had joined in this promising area of medical research and the benzodiazepine family had grown considerably.

The benzodiazepines – a much-needed solution

For badly trained, unprepared medical practioners suddenly facing an epidemic of mental disease, these drugs were an answer to many, if not all of their problems. The manufacturers' claims made it clear that the drugs were not only safe but that they were effective for just about all the problems doctors were likely to have to face. The inevitable result was that doctors greeted the new products with unbridled enthusiasm.

Within a year or two the benzodiazepines were among the most widely prescribed drugs in the world – with both Librium and Valium hitting the top of the best-selling drug charts around the world. For hospital doctors the benzodiazepines were a blessing and a boon. For general practioners they were a lifeline. With a prescription pad on his desk and a pen in his hand, a general practitioner could become a saviour to his patients.

Right from the start doctors found that their patients were happy to take Valium and similar drugs. The GP who happily prescribed the benzodiazepines without question would quickly become both popular and successful. The GP who was cautious about using the drugs would soon acquire a reputation for being rather difficult or mean. It was fashionable for doctors to prescribe the benzodiazepines. And it was quickly fashionable for patients to take them too.

By the early 1960s the drugs in this general category were being prescribed not only for straightforward anxiety states but also for a whole range of physical disorders. Shapiro and Bacon showed in 1961 that drugs in this group were being widely prescribed for patients with high blood pressure or with heart problems. They also reported that these drugs were being widely used for allergic, metabolic, respiratory, endocrine and nutritional conditions.

In 1962 Bacon and Fisher confirmed that doctors were prescribing these drugs for chest and heart problems but also added the information that they were using them for gastro-intestinal problems too.

As the years went by it became increasingly clear that doctors, particularly doctors in general practice, were using the benzo-diazepines to treat the whole range of physical and mental disorders known to be associated with stress, pressure and anxiety. Valium and its relatives had become the single answer to all the mental and physical manifestations of stress.

As their enthusiasm for Valium continued to grow many doctors started prescribing benzodiazepines in other rather inappropriate ways. So, for example, a survey done by Johnson and Clift in Manchester in 1968 showed that over half the patients started on night-time sedation with sleeping drugs were pre-scribed these pills because they were being kept awake by physical problems. Most of the patients, for example, were unable to sleep because of pain caused by problems such as arthritis, muscle pains and backache. It would, of course, have been far more appropriate to treat the cause of the sleeplessness rather than the insomnia itself.

Similarly it is difficult to understand why doctors used tranquillisers so often in the treatment of obesity, chronic bronchitis and other largely physical disorders.

It seems that the early success they had with Valium convinced many doctors that it was a universal panacea, suitable for all conditions known to man. So, when faced with a difficult diagnosis the doctor would reach for his prescription pad and scrawl the name of his favourite benzodiazepine.

The use of benzodiazepines is now so widespread that it is difficult to be dogmatic about just who is likely to receive a prescription for one of these drugs. It does seem, however, that anyone who visits a doctor with anything other than a single clear-cut request for specific treatment is likely to end up with a benzodiazepine. Visit your doctor with vague mental symptoms, with continuing aches and pains, or with any set of symptoms difficult to diagnose and the prescription you receive is likely to be for a benzodiazepine.

There is evidence too that many doctors (both male and female) exhibit signs of sexual discrimination when prescribing Valium. Over a dozen studies done in Europe, America, Canada and Australia, for example, have confirmed that women are far more likely to receive prescriptions for benzodiazepines than men. In particular it has been shown that women in their late forties, fifties and early sixties are extremely likely to be given pills in this group.

And where separate factors add together, then Valium becomes inevitable. A woman of fifty who goes to her GP with vague symptoms of any kind will almost certainly leave clutching a prescription for a benzodiazepine. Menopausal symptoms, insomnia, boredom, marital problems, aches and pains – the answer is the same.

Why did doctors accept the benzodiazepines so uncritically?
The thousands of doctors who suddenly started to prescribe Valium and so on in huge quantitites really knew very little about the drugs they were using. They simply accepted what they were told by the manufacturers.

There were two reasons for this incredible act of prescribing faith.

First, most doctors in practice today have grown up in a world where they are accustomed to getting their prescribing information from drug companies. For all doctors this is indeed the easiest way to keep up to date. A physician who qualified ten or more years ago will be quite out of touch with modern pharmacology, and won't understand a pharmacology journal even if he troubles to pick one up. If he isn't going to show his ignorance by using leeches and herb powders, then he has no option but to accept the easy-to-read brochures and leaflets from the drug company representatives and to accept the promises, claims and assertions printed on them. Even recently qualified doctors have to learn about new drugs in the same rather questionable way since medical schools treat pharmacology in much the same sort of way that they treat psychiatry – it is a very minor subject.

The second reason why doctors were happy to accept what they were told about the benzodiazepines was that they wanted to believe and needed to believe everything they read and heard. They desperately wanted the benzodiazepines to work. And so they never dreamt of questioning the promises and claims that were made.

As a result of their startling ignorance doctors in general practice commonly make mistakes when prescribing benzodiazepines. The most common errors are the following.

1. They allow patients to take Valium or some other drug in one of these groups for more than two months. This suggests clinical incompetence for two reasons. First the drug is known to be addictive and should, therefore, be used only for short-term problems. Second, the drug's efficiency drops as the weeks go by and after two months most patients taking a benzodiazepine will need to increase the dose in order to obtain any useful effect. (The increase in dosage may also be needed to disguise the symptoms produced by the drug itself, see page 74–75.) Third, the drug has no known clinical role in the treatment of long-term problems. It is a palliative and not a curative drug.

2. They prescribe in the wrong dosage. Because they get used to their chronic patients needing high doses of Valium, GPs will often prescribe those same high doses for new patients. This dangerous practice usually means that the patient suffers unduly from side effects. It also means that when the patient needs to increase his dosage in a month or two's time the daily intake must reach very high levels.

3. They mix benzodiazepines, often prescribing several drugs in this category for one patient. There isn't much point in this since there is little, if any, difference between the various available products.

37

4. They regularly use benzodiazepines for patients who can't get to sleep. Something like six per cent of the population of the United Kingdom take a sleeping tablet every night. In some hospitals the percentage of patients taking sleeping pills is very much higher – where pills are routinely handed out to all new patients the figure may get very close to 100 per cent.

But using sleeping pills as a long-term solution is both pointless and dangerous. It is pointless because there is now evidence to show that most sleeping pills work for no more than fourteen days. After that they lose their effectiveness and the dose needs to be increased for a similar effect to be obtained. And it is dangerous because there is also evidence to show that when a benzodiazepine sleeping pill is taken for a long period it can produce dependence.

What makes this ignorance particularly inexcusable is the fact that the hazards associated with the benzodiazepines have not been hidden but have been available to any doctor prepared to read anything other than drug-company sponsored publications.

So, for example, in a book called *Discoveries in Biological Psychiatry,* edited by Ayd and Blackwell, and published by Lippincott in 1970, Frank Ayd, then editor of the *International Drug Therapy Newsletter* wrote

'Although vast quantities of minor tranquillisers have been prescribed it must be stated that not all have been dispensed judiciously by some practitioners. Such misuse is indicative of physicians who unwisely accede to the demands of patients or who supplant sound clinical judgement for expediency. The disregard of these doctors for the potential abuse of minor tranquillisers and for the welfare of their patients is further manifested by their prescribing large quantities with no restrictions on refills and with no insistence that the patient return at regular intervals for evaluation of the response to or the need for the medication . . . these practices not only warrant condemnation but invite drug abuse. Clearly the abuse of some psychoactive drugs may call for the indictment of the physician and pharmacist rather than the drugs.'

Helped by the reaction against the barbiturates

Until the benzodiazepines came on to the market most doctors prescribed barbiturates for their anxious patients, for those patients who needed something to help them get to sleep, and for patients who just couldn't cope.

In the 1950s, however, it became clear that the barbiturates were neither safe nor suitable for widespread use. It became clear that they were addictive and dangerous drugs. In the early 1970s it was estimated that three people a day were dying from deliberate barbiturate overdosage alone.

All this bad publicity for the barbiturates meant that the introduction of the benzodiazepines was greeted with tremendous enthusiasm. Doctors who had for decades been happily prescribing barbiturates quickly changed their prescribing habits. Instead of dishing out barbiturates by the barrow load they dished out benzodiazepines by the barrow load.

Just how many benzodiazepines are there altogther?

When the World Health Organisation organised a seminar on psychotropic drugs (drugs that have an effect on the mind), in Moscow in 1979, it was estimated that there were approximately 1,000 drugs available which contained psychotropic ingredients. A great many of those were benzodiazepines. It has been estimated that there are about 700 Valium-like substances on the market.

The benzodiazepines are now almost certainly the most widely prescribed group of drugs in the world and the biggest selling drugs in the history of medicine. Over one billion dollars worth of benzodiazepines are sold each year.

Am I taking a benzodiazepine?

If you are taking any of the drugs named on this list (and the name of the drug you've been given should be on the bottle or packet you've been given) then you are taking a benzodiazepine. If you don't know what drug you've been given, then ask your doctor or pharmacist. You have a right to know what you are taking. This list is not, of course, complete.

The names which begin with a capital letter are branded names. Other names are chemical names.

Almazine	Frisium	Rohypnol
Alupram	Halcion	Serenid D
Anxon	ketazolam	Serenid Forte
Atensine	Lexotan	Solis
Ativan	Librium	Somnite
bromazepam	lorazepam	Stesolid
Centrax	lormetazepam	Surem
chlordiazepoxide	medazepam	temazepam
clobazam	Mogadon	**Tranxene**
clorazepate pot.	Nitrados	triazolam
Dalmane	nitrazepam	Unisomnia
diazepam	Nobrium	Valium
Euhypnos	Noctamid	Valrelease
Euhypnos Forte	Normison	Xanax
Evacalm	oxazepam	
flurazepam	**prazepam**	

The fact that a drug isn't on this list doesn't mean that it isn't a benzodiazepine. New products appear almost weekly and so no list can be completely up to date. If you are in any doubt about whether or not a drug that you are taking is a benzodiazepine, then ask your doctor. If he won't or can't tell you, then write to me c/o the publishers, telling me the name of the drug and I'll answer the question for you. Please note that you must send a stamped addressed envelope, and that I cannot offer advice about diagnosis or treatment.

Note
Most prescribed drugs are marked in some way. There is no standard system for this and the range of identifying marks is large, but with the aid of the appropriate reference books doctors and pharmacists can usually identify individual tablets and capsules with these letters and numbers.

In my view pills and capsules which carry no markings at all need to be treated with the same mixture of contempt and suspicion as anonymous letters. Any proud and responsible manufacturer who is confident that the quality of his product is good should be prepared to identify those tablets as his own.

If you visit a chemist and he dispenses unmarked tablets (or capsules) then I suggest that you cash your next prescription somewhere else. There is a risk that unidentifiable tablets may contain substantadard ingredients.

Are the many benzodiazepines different?

Doctors, pharmacists and researchers have been arguing for decades about whether or not there is any difference between the various benzodiazepines. Individual drug companies frequently claim special properties for their products. One company will say that its benzodiazepine has a particularly low incidence of side effects. Another will suggest that its product is especially good for patients who can't get to sleep. A third will suggest that it is the best drug for patients who are unable to relax.

When making these claims, drug companies will usually explain that the properties of different benzodiazepines depend upon molecular structure, possible dosage range, metabolic pathways and product half-life. (The product half-life enables observers to tell just how long a drug takes to pass through the body – some benzodiazepines have a long half-life and are effective for several days with the dosage accumulating as fresh pills are taken, while other benzodiazepines have much shorter half-lives and tend to be broken down and excreted from the body in a fairly short space of time.)

To support their claims, drug companies will usually point to published papers which provide apparent evidence supporting their assertions. The journals around the world are full of papers proving that this or that benzodiazepine is better than any others.

Sadly, these so-called research papers are not always as independent as they may appear to be, nor as significant as the drug companies quoting from them would like. For, in addition to the well established medical journals around the world there are also a number of other journals (often with very impressive names) which will publish papers for a fee. Such journals enable the drug companies to publish research work done for them by hired clinicians – and obviously the results of this type of work are likely to be favourable and laudatory.

The obviously and completely independent evidence which exists seem to show that in practice there is very little to choose between the different benzodiazepines. The British Committee on the Review of Medicines published a report in 1980 in which it stated that 'benzodiazepines are all equally effective in the short-term treatment of anxiety or insomnia; any classification of benzodiazepines as either anti-anxiety agents or hypnotics is unjustified'. The World Health Organisation's list of some 200 essential drugs lists only one benzodiazepine – diazepam.

Just about the only difference which does seem to exist between the benzodiazepines concerns their length of action in the body. So, for example, it seems that the benzodiazepines chlordiazepoxide, clorazepate, diazepam, flurazepam, medazepam and nitrazepam are all long-acting drugs suitable for patients needing longer-term treatment for anxiety (i.e. treatment lasting throughout the day). On the other hand lorazepam, oxazepam, temazepam and triazolam are all short-acting, and more suitable for patients requiring night-time sedation but not needing treatment for anxiety.

Even this difference seems, however, to be of very little significance. Some manufacturing drug companies seem to take little notice of whatever difference may exist and so we can, I think, safely assume that it is of no clinical value.

All the benzodiazepines can, therefore, be regarded as but one drug.

How popular are the benzodiazepines?

Tranquillisers are now used more regularly than all other classes of drugs. In Britain alone the current annual prescribing rate for tranquillisers is running at about fifty-five million prescriptions. Of these tranquillisers, the benzodiazepines are by far the most popularly prescribed group of drugs and Valium is the single most commonly prescribed benzodiazepine.

Valium is, probably, the single most commonly prescribed drug in the world – being top of just about every chart there is, and reaching a popularity in the pharmaceutical world that not even the Beatles or Elvis Presley ever reached in the world of pop music.

Valium is, in short, a pharmaceutical phenomenon.

42

The prescribing explosion still continues

Throughout the two decades after their introduction doctors continued to prescribe the benzodiazepines in greater and greater quantities. Beween 1965 and 1970 the number of prescriptions for drugs in this group rose steadily and by 1970 British GPs were writing over seventeen million prescriptions a year for tranquillisers. The benzodiazepines and other similar drugs made up approximately 6.5 per cent of all drugs prescribed by GPs. In other words if you went to see a GP in 1970 then you had a better than one-in-twenty chance that if you came away with a prescription it would be for Valium or something like it.

By 1975 the tranquillisers were even more popular with the total number of prescriptions for drugs in this category having reached forty-three million a year. One out of every six prescriptions written was for a drug in this general group.

Still the limits had not been reached. In 1977, the number of prescriptions reached forty-five million and a paper appeared in the *British Medical Journal* in which Richard Doll, Regius Professor of Medicine at the University of Oxford, D.C.G. Skegg, a lecturer in the epidemiology department, and J. Perry, the director of the Oxford Community Health Project, reported that psychotropic drugs accounted for almost one-fifth of all prescriptions with 9.7 per cent of the male population and 21 per cent of the female population receiving at least one of the drugs in this category during the year. For women in the forty-five to fifty-nine age group one in three were given a tranquilliser of some sort.

For twenty years the benzodiazepines have been the fastest growing prescription drug group in the world. There are no real signs of the explosion being reversed.

As the years have gone by more and more investigators have produced papers showing that the benzodiazepines are not as safe as was originally thought. On pages 49–69 of this book I have listed some of the evidence which shows the wide range of side effects and dangers associated with these drugs. Many of these research papers were first published ten or twenty years ago.

Despite this accumulation of damning evidence, however, many doctors continue to use the benzodiazepines as though they were as effective as the philosopher's stone and as harmless as chocolate drops. In countless naïve journal articles, doctors have displayed their ignorance with a remarkable lack of self-consciousness, often defending the use of the benzodiazepines as though they were a vital part of the modern doctor's therapeutic *armamentarium*.

And that, of course, is exactly what they are.

For the truth is that many doctors in practice today are addicted to prescribing these drugs. It's doctors, not patients, who are the worst addicts.

The benzodiazepines in hospitals

During the 1960s and 1970s the demand for medical attention continued to grow at a quite tremendous rate. Like their colleagues in general practice, hospital doctors began to consider the benzodiazepines to be a single answer to many problems. They were apparently safe drugs with few side effects.

One of the conditions for which the benzodiazepines had originally been recommended was insomnia and it is therefore hardly surprising that doctors in hospitals all over Britain took to routinely giving all new hospital patients a night-time dose of a benzodiazepine. The argument was that since going into hospital is a stressful event, patients are probably going to have difficulty in getting to sleep. Patients who stay awake at night are not only likely to be tired and sleepy the following day, but they are also likely to be a nuisance to the night staff.

So it became common practice for hospital patients to be given benzodiazepines routinely. And when the patient was discharged he was often given a bottle of sleeping pills to take with him – just to tide him over for the first few days at home.

When the discharged patient went to see his GP for a post-hospital check-up, the GP would provide a prescription for any treatment recommended by the hospital doctors. And the night-time sedation would be on that prescription.

In this simple way hundreds of thousand of people started taking benzodiazepines for the first time.

The benzodiazepines in general practice

As the number of people taking benzodiazepines continued to grow

44

doctors in general practice found themselves in a strange dilemma. They had originally started most of these patients on benzodiaze-pines because they didn't have the knowledge or time to deal with their problems more effectively. Valium was an immediate solution which helped to keep the flow of patients moving.

The problem was, however, that Valium didn't cure anyone. It kept some problems at bay and it numbed patients so that they didn't complain quite as much but it didn't solve anyone's problems or banish their symptoms. Consequently, general practitioners found that they had increased their own workload. All the patients who had been started on Valium or one of the other benzodiazepines wanted to come back for another appointment and another supply of pills.

GPs just couldn't cope. They did not have the time to deal with all these established patients. And so they started to provide more and more patients with 'repeat' prescriptions. In other words they allowed patients to collect a prescription for some pills without actually having to attend the surgery.

Now, in principle, it is reasonable to offer long-term patients repeat prescriptions. If you are a diabetic or epileptic there is no point in your attending the surgery every month to collect a prescription for your regular treatment. It saves everyone's time if the receptionist is instructed to accept requests from such patients for a fresh supply of their medication. Patients are simply instructed to ask for an appointment if they have any problems or unusual symptoms.

With the benzodiazepines, however, there was never any logical reason why patients should be able to collect repeat prescriptions. Valium and its associated drugs had never been recommended for long-term use. Even the drugs' makers claimed that it was best suited for short-term use. Valium is not a long-term drug.

Repeat prescriptions for benzodiazepines were introduced not because they were clinically sensible but because they were the only solution to a problem that doctors and patients could not otherwise solve. No doctor who had started more than a handful of his patients on benzodiazepins could hope to manage his practice unless he provided those patients with repeat prescriptions. And so today it is estimated that there are two million people in Britain who have taken a tranquilliser regularly for more than six months.

Thousands of GPs have become drug pushers and hundreds of thousands of their patients have become junkies.

One paper published in the *British Medical Journal* showed that one in ten of all patients receiving repeat prescriptions for drugs in this category had been receiving these pills for over ten years – some without seeing a doctor at all in that time. In practices where doctors insisted on seeing their patients every so often before providing repeat prescriptions the average time lapse between visits to the surgery was still nineteen weeks. These aren't figures relating to badly organised, elderly, drug-pushing doctors in poor inner-city practices. These are figures relating to ordinary British GPs.

As things are at the moment, the problem seems destined to get much worse before it gets any better. Instead of trying to work out ways to reduce the amount of repeat prescribing they do many doctors are, it seems, concentrating their efforts on looking for ways to simplify the process and make it easier to administer.

So, for example, in medical practices all over the country doctors are installing computers and using them to make it *even easier* for patients to obtain fresh supplies of drugs. With the aid of a computer, a specially written programme and a print-out a doctor can more or less isolate himself from the prescribing process. All he has to do is sign the prescription once the request has been processed and the form printed.

It is hardly surprising that the number of people taking benzodiazepines is growing year by year.

What of the future?

It is estimated that one in every three patients who visits a doctor has some sort of psychological problem. The potential profits to be made in this area are, therefore, quite vast. It is hardly surprising that many of the world's largest drug companies are spending huge amounts of money on looking for drugs that will have an effect on the mind, that will restore or even improve intellectual function, that will improve concentration or memory, or will simply act as safe and effective tranquillisers.

It is the search for the latter that is probably being pursued with the greatest enthusiasm. For, just as Roche succeeded in replacing the barbiturates when they introduced chlordiazepoxide and its relatives, so other drug companies, recognising that the problems with the benzodiazepines are rapidly frightening many patients and some prescribers, are searching for a new alternative. Roche made a fortune out of their discovery. The replacement for Valium will earn a fortune too. There are already companies working on non-benzodiazepine hypnotics and tranquillisers, said not to cause addiction of any kind.

I wonder if we are really all going to make the same mistake again. Ten years ago, in my first book, *The Medicine Men,* I predicted that doctors would end up trying to wean patients off the benzodiazepines. It seemed patently obvious at the time that Valium and its relatives would produce real problems, and that thousands of patients would get hooked.

I believe that in the next year or two we'll see a drug company producing an alternative to the benzodiazepines; a new, safer, tranquilliser. Again, I make the same prediction. Whatever the drug is, if it proves to be an effective tranquilliser, patients will get hooked on it. And in ten years' time we'll have the same problem once again.

Stresses and strains produce many problems but drugs are not the answer.

For many years barbiturates were regarded as useful, safe drugs for the treatment of insomnia, depression and all forms of anxiety. Then it was found that the barbiturates are dangerously addictive. Exactly the same pattern is now emerging with the benzodiazepines. And I believe that whatever pharmacological solution the drug companies may offer for mental problems of this kind, the drug they produce will be addictive.

Chapter 3.

DRAWBACKS AND HAZARDS

- The benzodiazepines and addiction
- The benzodiazepines and brain damage
- The benzodiazepines and memory capacity
- The benzodiazepines and anxiety or depression
- The benzodiazepines and aggression
- The benzodiazepines and the elderly
- The benzodiazepines and your sex life
- The benzodiazepines and driving
- The benzodiazepines and accidents at home and work
- The benzodiazepines and shoplifting
- The benzodiazepines and pregnancy
- The benzodiazepines and breast-feeding
- The benzodiazepines and tea or coffee
- The benzodiazepines and other drugs
- The benzodiazepines and cancer
- The benzodiazepines and your liver
- Miscellaneous side effects
- The effect of benzodiazepines on our society
- Just how dangerous are the benzodiazepines?
- Minor drugs?

The benzodiazepines and addiction

Although the numerous manufacturers producing and selling benzodiazepines make many different claims for their products, these drugs are fundamentally very similar. There really isn't as much difference between the various available products as the drug companies would like us all to believe.

So, for example, although Valium is sold for use as an anti-anxiety drug and Mogadon is sold as a sleeping pill, there is not much basic difference between the two substances. Doctors prescribe Valium for day-time use because they have been told to do just that. And they prescribe Mogadon as a sleeping tablet because that is what they have been told it is.

Because the basic constituents of these drugs are similar, the side effects and problems associated with them are similar too. So, each of the warnings and pieces of advice in this section can be applied to the majority of benzodiazepines currently available and likely to become available in the future.

In recent years the problem of benzodiazepine addiction has attracted an enormous amount of publicity. Numerous magazine and newspaper articles have been written on the subject and almost every time the subject has been mentioned the authors concerned have received hundreds of letters from men and women who have recognised that they have the same symptoms as the reported addicts. Doctors who have done radio phone-ins will confirm that if one caller rings up and talks about tranquilliser addiction the phone lines will usually become jammed with people complaining of identical symptoms.

Subjective reports like this are not scientific evidence, of course, and there are many who argue that the benzodiazepines do *not* cause addiction.

For two decades, for example, some people who make and sell the benzodiazepines have consistently argued that these drugs do not cause any such problems. They have been supported by a number of advisers and medical experts who have published papers extolling the virtues of this group of drugs. The whole question has been confused by the fact that there have been many discussions about what is meant by words such as 'addiction', 'dependence',

51

'tolerance', 'adaptation' and so on. The academic arguments about the meaning of these terms has often obscured the fundamental question of whether or not people who take Valium, and similar drugs, can get hooked.

My feeling is that in practice it doesn't matter whether people taking drugs simply develop a bad 'habit' or a physical 'dependence'. Nor does it make much difference whether they take increased doses because they have established a physical 'tolerance' to the drug or because they simply cannot manage without it.

After studying scores of existing research papers I am totally convinced that there is a *real* risk that anyone taking a benzodiazepine for more than a week or two will get hooked. And, moreover, I believe that the evidence in favour of the benzodiazepines producing dependence has been overwhelming for some years. The size of the addiction problem associated with these drugs has been regularly underestimated because most benzodiazepine addicts are allowed free access to supplies of the drug and the incidence of withdrawal symptoms has been consistently underestimated because relatively few individuals have tried to kick the benzodiazepine habit.

In support of my claim that the benzodiazepines *do* cause addiction I offer the following facts:

1. In 1975 three doctors from the Drug Dependence Treatment Center at the Philadelphia VA Hospital and University of Pennsylvania, Philadelphia, published a paper in *The International Journal of the Addictions* entitled 'Misuse and Abuse of Diazepam: An Increasingly Common Medical Problem'. Doctors Woody, O'Brien and Greenstein referred to papers published as far back as 1970 which had documented instances of physical addiction to chlordiazepoxide and diazepam and reported that since the end of 1972 they had noticed an increasing amount of diazepam misuse and abuse. Their paper concluded: 'All physicians should know that diazepam abuse and misuse is occurring and careful attention should be given to prescribing, transporting and storing this drug.'

2. In 1970 Dr Norman Imlah, Medical Director and Consultant Psychiatrist at All Saints Hospital, Birmingham, an expert on

drug addiction, published a book called *Drugs in Modern Society*. He wrote about the benzodiazepines: 'This is much too short a time to make a thorough assessment . . .' but went on to say that 'they are, however, regarded as very safe drugs, free from undesirable side reactions apart from a tendency to create dependence.'

So, even then, before the other side effects now associated with the benzodiazepines had been noted, it was clear that these drugs caused dependence.

3. In 1961, just a short time after chlordiazepoxide had been introduced into clinical practice, a clinical report appeared in *Psychopharmacologia* which was written by three physicians from the Veterans' Administration Hospital, Palo Alto, California. Entitled 'Withdrawal Reactions from Chlordiazepoxide ['Librium']', the paper described very dramatically how patients who had been taking the drug suffered from withdrawal symptoms when the drug was stopped.

The authors described how eleven patients who had been taking fairly high doses of chlordiazepoxide for up to six months were quite suddenly taken off the drug and given sugar tablets instead. Ten of the eleven patients experienced new symptoms or signs after the withdrawal of the chlordiazepoxide. Six patients became depressed, five were agitated and unable to sleep, two had major convulsions or fits. Most of the symptoms developed within two to nine days after the chlordiazepoxide was stopped, with most appearing between the fourth and the eighth days.

It is of course quite impossible to suffer withdrawal symptoms without being in some way addicted to a drug.

This report was, I repeat, published in 1961.

There are today, two decades later, doctors who *still* do not know that the benzodiazepines can cause addiction.

4. Testifying to a US Senate health sub-committee in Washington in 1979, a psychiatrist from a Californian rehabilitation unit claimed that patients can become hooked on diazepam in as little as six weeks. The same committee heard testimony that it is harder to kick the tranquilliser habit than it is to get off heroin. One expert witness said that tranquillisers provide America's number one drug problem apart from alcohol.

5. In a paper called 'Benzodiazepine Dependence', published in the *British Journal of Addiction* in 1981, Dr Petursson and Professor Lader of the Institute of Psychiatry in London reported that the 'benzodiazepines are fully capable of inducing both physical and psychological dependence'. They concluded their analysis of the problem by writing 'a careful examination of the problem . . . is a matter of urgency'.

6. In a symposium at the Royal Society of Medicine in April 1973, Dr John Bonn, at the time a senior lecturer and Consultant Psychiatrist at St Bartholomew's and Hackney Hospitals, London, said that 'The benzodiazepines are medications to be avoided, unless the patient is under close supervision.' He explained that he saw a number of benzodiazepine-dependent patients, and that when these patients were taken off their drugs they often felt much better than they had for years.

Despite the strength of this evidence the benzodiazepines are still easy to obtain. Doctors can prescribe them without any restrictions and although the drugs have been said to be even more addictive than drugs such as heroin they remain outside dangerous drug-control legislation.

One can but admire the power and effectiveness of the drug-industry lobby and their public relations and marketing advisers who have succeeded in persuading doctors to keep prescribing these drugs in huge quantities, and in persuading Government agencies to leave the drugs virtually outside the control of the law.

Ten years ago there was enough evidence to suggest that the availability of the benzodiazepines should be controlled by legislation. How much longer do we have to wait?

The benzodiazepines and brain damage

At a conference at the National Institute of Health in Washington, USA, in 1982, a British Professor of Psychopharmacology, Malcolm Lader, reported that brain scans done on a small group of patients who had been taking diazepam for a number of years had produced evidence suggesting that their brains had been damaged.

Although warning that his preliminary findings needed more research Professor Lader pointed out that the work he had done suggested that the brains of regular benzodiazepine takers were damaged and shrunken when compared to the brains of people who had not taken benzodiazepines.

There are no precise figures about the number of people who have taken diazepam for long periods of time, but Professor Lader calculates that something like 250,000 British people and over a million patients in America have taken tranquillisers for more than seven years – and could therefore have damaged brains.

I don't think anyone really knows what long-term effects the benzodiazepines are likely to have on brain tissue. But research reported at a neuropsychopharmacology congress in Jerusalem in 1982 suggested that the benzodiazepines may affect memory. Research has shown, for example, that volunteers who have taken benzodiazepines are unable to remember things like telephone numbers and map routes.

In addition to these suggestions that the benzodiazepines may damage your brain cells and produce real physical damage to your thinking processes, there is also the risk that the benzodiazepines will cause psychological damage. So, for example, there is the risk that while you are taking one of these drugs your emotional make-up will be dramatically changed. You may no longer suffer acute attacks of anxiety or depression while you are drugged. But, at the same time, you may also fail to enjoy the peaks of pleasure in your life. You may become 'zombie'-like in your attitude to life, and boring and uninteresting to those around you. As a result of these definite and obvious changes in your personality your relationships with other people may change. You may lose friends, you may lose your job and you may find that your marriage breaks up.

The benzodiazepines can affect your ability to think and your ability to enjoy life. They can have a powerful effect on your personality and on your relationships with the people closest to you too.

The benzodiazepines and memory capacity

In 1982 the Scandinavian *Journal of Psychology* published a paper entitled 'Amnesic Effects of Diazepam: "Drug Dependence" Explained by State-Dependent Learning'. The paper, written by two Danes, Hans Henrik Jensen of the University of Aarhus and Jens Christian Poulsen of the Psychiatric Hospital, Aalborg, described one of the most remarkable pieces of research to involve the benzodiazepines.

Jensen and Poulson began their work knowing that diazepam can produce amnesia for events which take place when the drug is being used. This effect is considered a useful bonus when diazepam is being utilised to sedate patients about to undergo surgery. The research done by Jensen and Poulson was designed to find out just how much patients on long-term diazepam treatments are affected by this phenomenon.

What they found was that if a patient takes diazepam he won't be able to remember things that he learned while taking the drug – unless he takes it again. This discovery is extremely important. For, as Jensen and Poulson imply, it suggests that if a patient learns to cope with his pressures and his problems and learns to relax and deal with external stresses while he is taking diazepam he will forget everything that he has learned when he stops taking the drug. As soon as he gives up his pills his memory will deteriorate so much that he'll forget all that he has learned about relaxing.

But if he then starts to take his diazepam again his memory will return. And he will, once more, be able to relax and deal with his pressure. He will feel comfortable and happy. Everything he has learned about how to cope without diazepam will be of value only when he is taking diazepam.

It's the ultimate Catch-22 situation.

And it is hardly surprising that diazepam, and the other benzodiazepines, are very difficult to give up!

The benzodiazepines and anxiety or depression

Diazepam and the other benzodiazepines are frequently prescribed for patients suffering from anxiety and mild depression. It is rather surprising, therefore, to discover that the benzodiazepines can actually *cause* these symptoms.

One report – published in 1972 in the *American Journal of Psychiatry* and written by Lt Cdr Richard C. W. Hall, MC, USN, and Joy R. Joffe, MD, when both were working at the Johns Hopkins University School of Medicine, Baltimore – described how six patients on diazepam had exhibited a cluster of symptoms which included tremulousness, apprehension, insomnia and depression. The patients had all been previously emotionally stable and the symptoms, which started suddenly, were quite severe. When these patients were taken off their diazepam their symptoms disappeared.

Other reports have confirmed the suggestion that the benzo-diazepines may produce anxiety rather than cure it. In Holland in 1979, for example, a psychiatrist contributed a paper to a Dutch medical journal in which he described how four patients taking a benzodiazepine sleeping tablet had developed severe anxiety and intolerable psychological changes. The report led to about 500 other, similar, complaints about the drug.

In 1982 a psychiatrist from the Royal Edinburgh Hospital, Edinburgh, reported that twenty-one middle-aged individuals who had been taking a benzodiazepine with a very short half-life to help them sleep had become slowly more anxious. Research suggested that even benzodiazepines thought to have a very short life in the body could produce noticeable anxiety for some time afterwards.

The really worrying thing about this research is perhaps that the link between the taking of benzodiazepines and the development of anxiety, although now well established by researchers, has still not been widely accepted by prescribing doctors. There are many general practitioners and hospital doctors who, when faced with anxious patients, will immediately write out prescriptions for benzodiazepines. Then, if their prescriptions don't seem to work and their patients become more anxious and more irritable, they will increase the dose.

In the light of the evidence now available this is difficult to explain.

In addition to this, there is now evidence to show that these drugs can also cause depression. There have been several such reports published but one of the earliest was perhaps the one published in the *Journal of the American Medical Association* in 1968. Most of the eight patients discussed in this research were taking diazepam in the normal dose of 5mg three or four times a day but the authors reported that their deepening depression was so severe that in seven patients suicidal thoughts and impulses occurred. Two of the patients are said to have made serious attempts to kill themselves while two succeeded.

Five of the patients showed improvements in three or four days after their diazepam was stopped.

No one really knows why there should be a link between the benzodiazepines and depression but could it be, perhaps, that when patients live exclusively in a dull, grey world where they are numbed and deprived of any peaks of pleasure, they drift very easily into despair and depression? Could it be that the benzodiazepines flatten emotions *too* effectively?

Finally, in this section I must point out that although those who favour the use of the benzodiazepines will often argue that these drugs are exceptionally safe when taken in large quantities the truth is that anyone who takes diazepam (or any other benzodiazepine) in large quantities is in real danger.

In one year in the early 1970s the number of deaths from diazepam (due either to suicide or accidental poisoning) reached sixteen in England and Wales alone. According to a paper published in the *Journal of the Royal Society of Medicine* in 1979, self-poisoning with tranquillisers, sleeping drugs and similar pills obtained on prescription accounts for 61,000 hospital admissions each year.

From the evidence which is available to us it seems that the benzodiazepines are not suitable for use by anxious, depressed or suicidal patients.

The benzodiazepines and aggression

When they were first introduced into clinical practice in the early 1960s both chlordiazepoxide and diazepam were publicly acclaimed for their ability to quiet, calm and tame wild animals. Because of these early animal experiments it was assumed that these drugs would have a similarly calming effect on human beings.

However, the research that was done in the 1960s did not really support this hypothesis. There was, to say the least, much confusion.

So, for example, although Kalina in 1964 gave diazepam to fifty-two prisoners and later reported that he had obtained complete control of violent, destructive and anti-social behaviour, Kelly and Giavold in 1960 found that chlordiazepoxide had the opposite effect.

And while Gleser in 1965 showed that male delinquents could be made less hostile with chlordiazepoxide, Feldman in 1962 had found that diazepam not only had no favourable effect on the hostility of patients, but that in many cases patients' hates became more, and not less, intense.

Other workers too found that the benzodiazepines seemed to increase hostility, aggressiveness and irritability, making patients more self-assertive than usual.

One researcher who had studied the question of aggressiveness caused by benzodiazepines was Alberto DiMascio of the Department of Mental Health at the Commonwealth of Massachusetts and Tufts University School of Medicine, Boston. In 1975 he published a paper in *Psychopharmacologia* entitled 'The Effects of Benzodiazepines on Aggression. Reduced or Increased?' in which he summarised the conflicting evidence and suggested that before doctors could know for sure whether a benzodiazepine they were prescribing would cause more or less aggression more research would be needed.

For a while the problem of whether or not the benzodiazepines could have an effect on human aggression was the subject of some controversy within the medical journals. In 1975, for example, the *British Medical Journal* published an editorial entitled 'Tranquillisers Causing Aggression' in which the author recalled that way back in 1960 two authors writing in *The Lancet* had reported that a patient taking chlordiazepoxide had physically assaulted his wife for the first time in their twenty years of marriage.

It was also pointed out that the sort of people most likely to become hostile when taking benzodiazepines were those subject to frustration, and the author of the editorial concluded that 'If these are valid conclusions then they provide clear evidence that there may be dangers in the growing practice of prescribing minor tranquillisers for anxiety and tension brought about by environmental frustration and disturbed inter-personal relationships.'

Other doctors have agreed with that conclusion. It has, for example, been suggested that there is a link between baby battering and tranquillisers. Young mothers, it is said, take benzodiazepines because they cannot cope with their babies' demanding behaviour. But the behaviour doesn't change and nor does the environment. The drugs makes the mothers more aggressive – and when the baby cries again it is battered.

Despite this evidence the benzodiazepines are still widely used for people under pressure. The current baby-battering epidemic which is causing so much concern may well be a result of doctors over-prescribing these drugs.

The benzodiazepines and the elderly

When a 75-year-old lady was admitted to hospital in Newcastle upon Tyne in the early 1970s she was unable to walk or speak clearly, and was confused and incontinent – in short, in quite a dreadful state. The old lady had been taking a 5mg tablet of nitrazepam every night for at least a year.

Perhaps remembering that in the past doctors had had considerable success with similarly afflicted patients by stopping their bromide or their barbiturate tablets, the geriatricians at the Newcastle General Hostpial simply stopped the sleeping pill. Three days later the old lady was completely her old self.

After this and a number of similar experiences two specialists in the treatment of the elderly in the Department of Geriatric Medicine at the Newcastle General Hospital wrote a letter to the *British Medical Journal* which was published in November 1972. They pointed out that 'despite statements to the contrary made in advertising literature, nitrazepam seems a particularly unsuitable hypnotic for old people.' They reported that they were seeing no less than six or seven similar cases every month and suggested that the drug no longer be used for elderly patients.

In the years which followed that report several other journals have published articles telling much the same story, and geriatricians in many areas have stopped using benzodiazepines for elderly patients.

Unhappily, general practioners don't very often read journal articles or letters – they get most of their prescribing information from drug-company representatives, advertisements and colleagues in general practice – and so the benzodiazepines have continued to be widely prescribed for elderly patients.

Reports are still continually published in the journals describing the same sort of problems as those initially described back in 1972 by those perspicacious geriatricians in Newcastle upon Tyne.

The benzodiazepines and your sex life

It has been known for centuries that drugs such as alcohol can increase sexual desire but, at the same time, have an adverse effect on sexual performance. Alcohol can make you randy, but it can also prove sadly disabling.

There is evidence too that the benzodiazepines can have a similarly sad effect. I don't think anyone knows the extent of any such relationship and I certainly have not been able to find any evidence showing that benzodiazepines have any effect on the brain or the pathways which carry sexual impulses from the brain to the parts that matter.

But it certainly seems possible that the depression sometimes caused by benzodiazepines can produce a fall in sexual desire and a drop in performance quality too. The numbing effect of these drugs can have a sad result too – one man, for example, reported that he had difficulty in getting an erection while taking Librium. Sometimes, according to Patricia J. Bush in *Drugs, Alcohol and Sex,* he just couldn't ejaculate at all.

The benzodiazepines and driving

There have, over the years, been a number of studies done which have shown that there is a link between the taking of benzodiazepines and road accidents.

One of the most impressive reports was, however, the one written by Professor Doll, Dr Skegg and Dr Richards of the University of Oxford, and published in the *British Medical Journal* in 1979. For this paper Skegg, Richards and Doll looked at the records involving over 40,000 people and compared prescriptions provided by general practitioners with records of road accidents, hospital admissions and deaths. They found a 'highly significant association between the use of minor tranquillisers and the risk of a serious road accident'. The risk of being involved in a serious accident is five times greater if you are taking a benzodiazepine than it is if you are not.

In another study, this time done in Holland, nine police driving instructors were given diazepam tablets and instructed to undertake a driving test. After taking a modest dose of 10mg the drivers 'seemed unable to maintain a straight course'.

A third survey showed that drivers who take a benzodiazepine at night to help them sleep will be affected if they sit behind a car steering wheel the following morning.

There have been dozens of such studies around the world, and authors in the United States of America, Finland, Norway and New Zealand have all confirmed the link between traffic accidents and drugs of this kind.

There have been some strong statements on the subject in Australia too. In 1981 the *Medical Journal of Australia* published an article by Landauer who argued that people taking diazepam need not avoid car driving. He argued that diazepam relieves anxiety, aggression and depression, and that its consumption need not, therefore, preclude motor car driving. In January 1982, however, the same journal published a paper by R. F. Soames Job, a behavioural scientist with the Traffic Accident Research Unit in New South Wales, Australia, who countered Landauer's arguments and suggested that the effect of diazepam on driving skills and ability is so great that anyone who takes the drug should avoid all driving.

Indeed, Mr Job points out that driving in Australia while under the influence of diazepam is an offence. It seems reasonable to point out that the same is also true of most other countries. It would probably be difficult to define that phrase accurately but I suppose it is fair to say that anyone whose reactions, muscular coordination or mental state had been affected by a drug could be described as 'under the influence'. Since there is simple evidence that diazepam affects these responses, any individual shown to have a measurable level of diazepam in his blood could be prosecuted.

In the February 1983 edition of the *Adverse Drug Reaction Bulletin*, Dr Heather Ashton, MA, DM, FRCP, Honorary Consultant in Clinical Pharmacology to Newcastle Health Authority and Senior Lecturer in Pharmacology at the University of Newcastle, points out that between 11 and 20 per cent of drivers involved in traffic accidents were taking tranquillisers, that benzodiazepines impair performance and coordination, and that at least one recent report has suggested that people who drive for a living should never be allowed to take benzodiazepines.

From the conclusive evidence available it is now quite clear that no one taking any benzodiazepine should be allowed to drive or ride *any* sort of vehicle – whether it be a bus, train, taxi, car or motor cycle.

While millions of people take drugs like Valium and drive motor cars, the risks to everyone must be colossal. The number of people driving under the influence of drugs probably exceeds the number driving under the influence of alcohol. It seems bizarre and inexplicable that we should stop people driving when they have been drinking alcohol but allow them to drive when they have taken benzodiazepines.

My view is that anyone who drives within forty-eight hours of taking any benzodiazepine is behaving irresponsibly. Perhaps if insurance companies were to refuse to pay claims made by drivers who had had accidents after taking benzodiazepines then public opinion would change. Meanwhile, many more innocent pedestrians, cyclists and drivers must no doubt be killed before the laws on drug taking and driving are revised.

The benzodiazepines and accidents at home and work

The benzodiazepines slow down reaction times and they produce drowsiness. It is these effects which make these drugs so dangerous for the individual thinking of driving a motor car.

The risks are not confined to drivers, however. Anyone who operates machinery or whose job or occupation involves delicate, potentially dangerous work needs to take extra care when taking one of these drugs. If you operate sharp or fast-moving machinery, if you use food mixers, if you need to cook or heat food, if your job takes you up steps or ladders, or if you do anything else where you need fine movements and good reflexes then you should take extra special care if you are taking a benzodiazepine.

A spate of accidents could suggest that the drug you are taking is endangering your health – even your life.

The benzodiazepines and shoplifting

If you have ever walked through a supermarket, picked something up and accidentally put it into your bag or pocket, then you'll know how easy it is for an innocent shopper to find himself or herself on a shoplifting charge. The many tricks used by supermarket owners to encourage customers to pick up things they don't really want work very well. And by the time they reach the check-out desk many shoppers will be in a light trance.

All these problems are increased, and the dangers exacerbated when a shopper is taking a benzodiazepine. Drugged and drowsy, numb and forgetful, the shopper's chances of being arrested for shoplifting are magnified many times.

Anyone taking a benzodiazepine, or any other tranquilliser or sleeping pill, should be particularly careful when shopping. Try to get out of the shop as soon as possible – and if at all practicable don't go shopping alone.

The benzodiazepines and pregnancy

There is a risk of damage to your unborn baby if you take a benzodiazepine during a pregnancy. If you take a benzodiazepine at the start of your pregnancy then there is a risk that the baby will be born deformed. (Researchers have, for example, shown an increased incidence of babies born with cleft palates among women who have taken diazepam during pregnancy.) And if you take a benzodiazepine at the end of your pregnancy then there is a risk that your baby will have difficulty in surviving the traumas of birth.

The benzodiazepines and breast-feeding

Although some doctors prescribe benzodiazepines for mothers who are breast-feeding, this is a possibly dangerous practice. The benzodiazepines may be passed on in the breast milk and then absorbed by the feeding infant. There is still not much evidence to show what dangers exist.

In January 1983 the editors of the *Drug and Therapeutics Bulletin* pointed out that 'drowsiness and poor feeding occur with regular use of high doses of benzodiazepines'.

The benzodiazepines and tea or coffee

Most of us don't think of caffeine as a drug. It is, however, a fairly powerful stimulant which has a considerable effect on many parts of the human body. And it is, of course, present in fairly large quantities in such common drinks as tea and coffee.

Many of the people who drink tea and coffee (and who therefore take regular supplies of caffeine) also use one or other of the benzodiazepines. Recently, doctors have become worried by this massive simultaneous consumption of two fairly powerful drugs, and they have tried to find out just what sort of effect the two drugs may have when used together.

Downing and Rickels of the Psychopharmacology Research and Treatment Unit, Department of Psychiatry, University of Pennsylvania, Philadelphia, USA, have reported that 'particular substances contained in coffee and tea . . . stimulate the synthesis of hepatic enzymes which metabolise . . . benzodiazepines'.

In practical terms it has been shown that fairly modest doses of caffeine (two or three cups of coffee are enough) can counteract the effect of a dose of benzodiazepine.

Mattila, Palva and Savolainen of the Department of Pharmacology at the University of Helsinki, Finland, have shown in experiments with medical students (reported in the journal *Medical Biology* in 1982), that the calming effect of diazepam is counteracted by caffeine.

This all means that anyone taking a benzodiazepine and also drinking more than two cups of tea or coffee is likely to increase the benzodiazepine dose he is taking in order to obtain a useful effect. It also means that the strain on the body's metabolic pathways is likely to be very high.

Incidentally, for the record, it is perhaps also worth noting that Downing and Rickels showed that substances contained in cigarette smoke also have an effect on the way that the benzodiazepines are metabolised. It is difficult to be dogmatic about the possible consequences when cigarettes, coffee and benzodiazepines are mixed!

The benzodiazepines and other drugs

Like all drugs the benzodiazepines work by having an effect on the organs and tissues of your body. Their main effect is on your brain but they get there by travelling in your bloodstream and therefore they can (and must) reach every part of your body on their travels.

All this means that if you take a benzodiazepine and another drug then there may be a risk of an unhappy, even dangerous interaction. It would be impossible to list here all the possible hazards but I have listed below some of the most important interactions that can take place.

I can't tell you exactly what will happen – in most cases no one really knows – but benzodiazepines don't mix with:

  alcohol
  barbiturates
  antacid mixtures for indigestion and ulcer pains
  cimetidine (Tagamet), the anti-ulcer drug
  anti-diabetic drugs
  levadopa (for Parkinson's disease)
  anti-depressants
  anti-epilepsy drugs
  anti-coagulants
  thyroid drugs
  anti-histamines (for allergy reactions, hay fever etc)
  anaesthetics
  caffeine (in tea, coffee, cola drinks)

The benzodiazepines and cancer

For several years now there has been a simmering controversy about whether or not diazepam can cause cancer.

The first report to arouse real interest appeared in the form of a letter written to the editor of *The Lancet* in 1979 by Horrobin, Ghayur and Karmali of the Clinical Research Institute of Montreal, Canada. They reported that their research with animals had suggested that diazepam could have tumour-promoting properties. In other words, although it did not directly cause cancer, it could make a growth develop in individuals already susceptible to cancer.

66

In addition to pointing out that tranquillisers might accelerate tumour growth in human beings Horrobin, Ghayur and Karmali also complained that four applications for funds for more studies had been turned down.

After Horrobin announced his findings in public he was, he claims, 'forced out of his research position at the University of Montreal'. At a meeting of the American Association for the Advancement of Science in 1981, however, he repeated his suggestion that diazepam might be linked to cancer and pointed to a British study which had linked cancer growth to anxiety. Horrobin argued that the women whose breast cancers had developed more quickly had been taking diazepam and he suggested that more research was needed in order to clarify the position.

His work was never conclusive (although other researchers produced supporting evidence), but neither was his hypothesis ever disproved.

So, no one can tell you for certain whether benzodiazepam causes cancer. It may be that women who are anxious and therefore more likely to take tranquillisers are more likely to get cancer. It may be that Horrobin's initial work was wrong. And that the other researchers were wrong too. It may be that if you take these drugs then you are more likely to develop cancer.

No one knows for sure. And the benzodiazepines are still the most widely prescribed drugs in the world.

The benzodiazepines and your liver

In May 1982 a report appeared in Vol. 27, No. 5 of *Digestive Diseases and Sciences* in which Francis J. Tedasco, MD, and Luther R. Mills, MD – of the Department of Medicine, Section of Gastroenterology at the Medical College of Georgia, Augusta, Georgia, USA, and the Department of Pathology at the same college – outlined evidence showing that diazepam can cause liver damage.

Their evidence seems to me to prove quite conclusively that diazepam can cause direct liver damage when taken by mouth in a normal dose. What damage is likely to be caused by the long-term consumption of diazepam is not known.

Tedasco and Mills were so impressed by their findings that they concluded their article with the suggestion that, 'the widespread usage of this drug necessitates closer evaluation of liver-function tests while patients are receiving this drug'.

In practical terms this suggests that patients currently taking diazepam should be having regular liver tests done.

Miscellaneous side effects

Many other side effects have been reported by patients using benzodiazepines and by doctors prescribing them. Low blood pressure, visual disturbances, intestinal problems, skin rashes, bladder disorders, headaches, confusion, dizziness, blood diseases and allergy difficulties are just some of the named side effects.

In the period from January 1964 to February 1982 the Committee on Safety of Medicines in London received reports about well over 100 *different* side effects said to have been related to the use of diazepam alone. Other benzodiazepines produced their own fearfully impressive lists of side effects.

The effect of benzodiazepines on our society

Throughout Europe and America, and indeed the whole of the 'civilised world', a number of surveys have been done in an attempt to find out just how many people take tranquillisers. And the figures usually show that something like 10 per cent of the male population and 15 per cent of the female population are fairly regular users. In some parts of the world the figures are way above these – they are rarely much below. World-wide sales of the benzodiazepines are worth in excess of one billion dollars a year.

Quite apart from the risks to individual consumers of these tablets, capsules and medicines there is, I believe, an enormous risk to our society. Individuals who take benzodiazepines become numbed and easily moulded, they tend to accept things without protest, and they feel little in the way of emotional responses. That's the way the benzodiazepines work – they turn anxious, worried human beings into zombies. Giving up the drugs is difficult because it means being exposed to a whole range of frightening and disturbing stimuli. The benzodiazepine user gets hooked because life *with* Valium is comfortable and undemanding.

This state of affairs suits the politicians and bureaucrats as much as it suits the drug companies. A docile and uncomplaining population is easy to manage and administer.

It's not quite the way that Orwell saw it happening. But the end result is the same.

Just how dangerous are the benzodiazepines?

It's difficult to be specific about 'risk' factors but on the available evidence I think that if you are looking for a crutch and you intend to choose between tobacco and the benzodiazepines then you'll probably be better off choosing tobacco.

The risks associated with tobacco have been well described and explained in close detail by many experts. Cigarettes cause cancer, heart disease and chest problems. But if you need something to help you get through life and you want to choose between a cigarette and a Valium tablet then I would recommend the cigarette.

I think that doctors would serve some anxious patients better if they gave them prescriptions for filter cigarettes rather than benzodiazepines.

Minor drugs?

When accused of over-prescribing the benzodiazepines many doctors defend their actions by describing the drugs in this group as 'minor tranquillisers'. The term has, indeed, been accepted by many professional health-care experts and outside observers as though it had some significance and as though it justified the abuse of these drugs by doctors.

The truth is that the benzodiazepines are not 'minor' in any way. They are prescribed in huge quantitites, they have very noticeable side effects, and they are potentially hazardous.

The wide use of this deprecatory phrase has contributed to the abuse of the benzodiazepines.

Chapter 4.

ADDICTION AND KICKING THE HABIT

- How to tell if you're hooked
- Why you should kick the habit
- How to kick the habit
- Beware

How to tell if you're hooked

Answer these questions:

Have you been taking a benzodiazepine for three months or longer?
Yes/No

Have you needed to increase your dose of benzodiazepine since you first started taking it?
Yes/No

Has your doctor changed your brand of benzodiazepine?
Yes/No

Do you still have any of the symptoms for which you originally took a benzodiazepine?
Yes/No

Have any of your original symptoms got worse?
Yes/No

Do you obtain your benzodiazepines on repeat prescriptions?
Yes/No

Do you permanently suffer from drowsiness, tiredness, lethargy or unsteadiness?
Yes/No

If you miss a benzodiazepine when you would normally take one do you suffer any unusual symptoms?
Yes/No

Do you have to carry your benzodiazepines around with you?
Yes/No

Do you worry if your supply of benzodiazepines gets low?
Yes/No

If you have answered YES to any of these questions you *may* be hooked on Valium (or whatever benzodiazepine you are taking). You will need to cut your consumption of the drug slowly and carefully.

Why you should kick the habit

Some benzodiazepine addicts claim that they need their pills in order to cope with life. They argue that without drugs such as Valium they would not be able to deal with everyday problems, they would not be able to get to sleep, and they would not be able to relax. Most important of all they claim that they and they alone should have the right to decide whether or not to take their Valium, Librium, Mogadon or whatever. They argue that it is their life and they are entitled to do whatever they like with it.

These are, of course, the standard arguments put forward by all addicts. Exactly the same claims are made by coffee drinkers, cigarette smokers, alcoholics, heroin addicts, cocaine addicts and all other individuals dependent on drugs.

The truth about the benzodiazepines is, however, that they do not help relieve either insomnia or anxiety when taken for long periods of time. Numerous researchers have shown that none of the drugs in this group work for more than a matter of weeks. Indeed, on the contrary, after they have been taken for some weeks all the benzodiazepines tend to produce the very symptoms they were originally taken to quell.

Kicking the habit – and giving up benzodiazepines – is quite likely to lead to an improvement of the symptoms for which the benzodiazepines were themselves being taken.

How to kick the habit

If you are hooked on a benzodiazepine then you will need to wean yourself off the drug with care and caution. Read the following notes carefully and keep this book somewhere handy so that you can read them again whenever things are not going well.

1. When you stop taking a benzodiazepine you may experience unpleasant symptoms. The most common symptoms are these:

    Tremor and shaking
    Intense anxiety – sometimes a feeling of panic
    Dizziness and giddiness

A feeling of faintness
An inability to get to sleep and an inability to sleep through the
    night
An inability to concentrate properly
Nausea
A metallic taste in the mouth
Depression
Headaches
Clumsiness and poor coordination
Increased sensitivity to noise, light and touch
A feeling of tiredness and lethargy
A feeling of 'being outside your body'
Blurred vision
Hot and cold feelings and a burning on your face
Aching muscles
An inability to speak normally
Hallucinations
Confusion
Sweating
Fits

You may suffer one or more of these symptoms when you stop taking your benzodiazepine. The symptoms will usually start a day or two after you have stopped taking the drug and will usually continue for up to three weeks afterwards.

The withdrawal symptoms can be minimised by reducing your dose slowly and enabling your body to accustom itself to life without the drug. The rate at which you reduce your dosage of benzodiazepine will depend upon the size of the dosage you have been taking. As a rule of thumb you should halve your dose every two weeks until it can no longer be halved.

So, for example, if you are taking two benzodiazepines every evening cut down to one every evening for a fortnight and then to half a tablet every evening for another fortnight. Then cut the drug out altogether.

If you are taking more tablets each day then you can cut your daily dosage more gently. So, for example, if you take six tablets a day you can reduce to five tablets a day for four days, then to four tablets a day for another four days, then to three tablets a day for another four days. That will mean that you will have halved your initial dose in about two weeks.

Obviously, the higher the dose of drug you are taking the longer it will take you to wean yourself off the drugs altogether.

3. If you originally took your benzodiazepine for anxiety then the chances are that when you stop the drug your original symptoms will return. If you originally took your benzodiazepine because you could not get to sleep then the chances are that when you stop the drug you will once again have difficulty in getting to sleep.

Benzodiazepines don't cure anything – they merely hide symptoms.

Clearly, therefore, when you stop taking your benzodiazepine you are going to have to learn how to cope with your anxiety or sleeplessness in some other way. I suggest that before you start to cut down your benzodiazepines you read pages 79–107 of this book and start putting the advice there into practice.

4. Your attempts to wean yourself off your benzodiazepines will not succeed unless you genuinely want to stop taking the drug. The first few days without the drug will be uncomfortable and unpleasant.

If, however, you want to manage without the drug then you will be able to kick the habit. And afterwards you will almost certainly feel much better than you have for some time.

5. Do not take any other drugs, tablets or medicines brought from the chemist to help you over the period of withdrawal. And do not allow well-meaning friends to give you pills to help you through the difficult days. Do not use alcohol as a crutch either.

6. You should warn your friends and family that you are likely to be going through a tricky few days. Tell them what to expect and explain that you would welcome a little extra support, sympathy and patience. The chances are that among your friends you will find someone else who is also taking a benzodiazepine and who also wants to 'kick the habit'. If the two of you decide to give up your drugs together then you can

lean on each other. Ring one another up, keep in touch, share your problems, and keep your determination alive.

7. Don't try and give up benzodiazepines if you are going through a particularly difficult patch (if, for example, you are moving house or coping with unusual problems at work). Wait until things are a little more settled before you try to give up your pills.

8. Before you begin your 'withdrawal' period you should visit your doctor and tell him what you plan to do. Ask him to help you.

Beware

When you try giving up your benzodiazepines you will probably feel anxious and rather miserable. You may have other symptoms – such as the ones on the list on pages 74–75.

If you visit your doctor and tell him that you have acquired these symptoms since giving up your tranquilliser he will probably suggest that you start taking your tablets again. He might point out that you were better when you were taking the pills, and that you obviously need some support. If he hasn't read the medical literature for a decade or two he will probably assure you that the benzodiazepines are not dangerous or addictive.

If you follow his advice then you will probably succeed in getting rid of your immediate withdrawal symptoms.

But you'll be back on your benzodiazepines.

And you'll be hooked again.

Chapter 5.

LIVING WITH ANXIETY

- Coping without tranquillisers
    - Coping with guilt
    - Coping with boredom
    - Coping with vanity
    - Coping with frustration
    - Coping with ambition
    - Coping with fear
    - Coping with lust
- Recognise your early-warning signs
- Learn to cope with anxiety or panic attacks
- Everything you need to know about getting to sleep
- Relax your body
- Relax your mind
- Take a break
- Remember the values of organisation
- The escape clause
- Remember that depression and anxiety can be contagious
- Rock away the blues
- Let your emotions show

Coping without tranquillisers

Our modern lifestyle produces many stresses and strains, and every day millions of people will continue to find their thresholds being breached. The benzodiazepines have undoubtedly provided many of us with a useful, short-term solution. Without these drugs we have to look for other answers, other solutions.

In this last section of this book I have outlined some of the ways that I have found effective in helping patients cope with pressure. You won't need to try all these solutions – you may find that some of them sound impractical or unsuitable. But read through these pages and use the advice they contain to help put together a survival programme of your own.

Earlier in this book, on pages 9–23, I described the seven deadly driving forces – pressures which I believe lead to anxiety and tension and which are often responsible for the initial need for tranquilliser support. If you read those pages again you should be able to see which forces have most effect on your life – here, on the pages which follow, you'll find advice on just how to cope with each of these destructive forces. You must first of all identify which factors are causing your stress – and then do something about them.

Coping with guilt

1. You must first of all decide whether you feel guilty because you *have* done something wrong or because you *feel* that you have done something wrong, perhaps because you have let down someone close to you or someone whose expectations you have failed.
2. If you have done something clearly and obviously wrong (damaged a parked car, broken a plate or whatever), then you must accept responsibility for your deed and with that responsibility you must accept whatever penalties may be involved. Once your potential feelings of guilt have been assuaged in this practical way then you can try and learn from the incident. If, for example, you had a minor car accident then it may be that you were rushing because you were late.

Perhaps you could avoid future problems of a similar kind by setting out a little earlier next time. When the guilt is easily defined then the solution is fairly easy to define.

3. When your guilt has been produced not by an easily defined crime or wrong-doing but by a nebulous feeling of having failed in some way then the chances are that you feel guilty because someone else has made you feel that way. There is no wrong that you can right, no error that you can repair, and no way that you can learn from your experience.

This is the sort of guilt that causes most pain and to deal effectively with it you must find and isolate the cause. Try to decide precisely why you feel so guilty. Do you feel that you have failed your parents, a friend, your employer, your children or your God? Before you can begin to deal with your guilt you must isolate and identify the cause.

4. Much of the guilt we suffer is produced by those who are closest to us. So in order to protect yourself a little you must learn to differentiate between the realistic and sensible expectations of those who are near to you and the purely selfish expectations they may harbour. Identify the people who are likely to make unreasonable demands on you and make it clear to them that you are not prepared to put your conscience at their disposal. Define your own ambitions, your own moral standards and your own boundaries of reasonable responsibility and the make it clear to those around you that you are not prepared to feel guilty every time you fail to satisfy the aspirations and expectations of other individuals or groups.

5. Don't put too many demands on yourself and don't let anyone else put too many demands on you either. Whatever it is that you have done wrong and whatever it is that you are feeling guilty about you should remember that you are only human and that human beings have a tendency to make mistakes.

When you have done something worth feeling guilty about then you should do all that you can to repair the damage, you should do your best to ensure that you learn from the experience and that you minimise the chance of there being another error of the same kind. That's all that you – or anyone else – can expect.

6. If you find yourself punishing yourself endlessly and un-reasonably for something you have done, try to imagine how you would feel if someone else had done what you have done. Try to see yourself as an impartial observer. Would you be as hard on them as you are being on yourself? Would you forgive them? Compassion, like charity, should begin at home. Be fair to yourself.

7. Don't put up with people who keep making you feel guilty. Make it clear to them that you are not prepared to put up with their demands on your conscience. Anyone who consistently makes you feel guilty is stupid, greedy, selfish or wicked. No one has a right to make others suffer and anyone close to you who consistently makes you feel guilty does not deserve your friendship.

8. Try to put your guilt into perspective. Will your guilt still be justified in ten years' time? Will your evil deeds still look quite so black? Try to imagine how significant your wrong-doings will appear in another decade. Try to figure out how big a part they will have played in your life and the lives of those who are dearest to you. This perspective test is often very telling. You'll be surprised how often something that seems to be extremely important will turn out to be relatively trivial.

9. To others you are a mother, a wife, a girlfriend, an employee, an employer, a daughter, a nurse, an assistant or a friend. But never forget that you have rights as an individual too. To other people you may fulfil a particular role in their lives – but don't let that impinge on your own right to enjoy your life. You have a right to some freedom of your own. You have a right to make some decisions without always thinking of other people. You have a right to expect others to treat you as an individual with feelings, emotions, needs and desires.

To deal effectively with guilt you must get the right balance between your responsibilities, your conscience, your love for those close to you, your willingness to please, and your own rights and responsibilities as an individual.

If you are the sort of person who suffers a lot from guilt then the chances are that you are also the sort of person who doesn't pay too much attention to your own feelings. Don't let your personality be suffocated by guilt inspired by others.

10.　Don't underestimate yourself or underrate yourself. If you are the sort of person who suffers a lot from guilt then you probably have a lot to be proud of. Guilt-ridden individuals tend to be honest, hard-working, generous, gentle and conscientious. Sit down with a piece of paper and a pencil and write down all the good things about yourself. Don't be modest. Imagine that you are writing your own obituary and you are trying to pick out all your good points. Then try to pick out all your bad points. If you have been honest and fair to yourself then you will almost certainly find that the good points far outweigh the bad points.

So, take a little pride in yourself. You probably have far more going for yourself than you have ever realised before. You could perhaps benefit by being a little more selfish from time to time.

Coping with boredom

1.　If you find your job boring, whether in a factory or at home, try and look for ways to make it more interesting. If it entails a series of routine tasks, look for ways that those tasks can be speeded up or simplified. Think of ways in which your productivity can be improved or the quality of your product enhanced. This can apply equally well to the production line or dusting!

2.　If your daily work brings you face to face with machinery of any kind then do your best to find out just how that machinery works. Ask for instruction manuals and read them. Write to the manufacturers for background information and any details that you can't find. If you master a machine it will become your servant instead of your nightmare. You will find that you will be able to mend it yourself, you will know what mechanics and repairmen are talking about when they say that the 'tappit-hinge bracket needs reboring' and you'll find your daily work far less boring.

3.　Even if a daily job is irretrievably boring you can add excitement and fun to your life by taking up a hobby which you find rewarding. It doesn't matter whether it is gardening, breeding canaries, making models of the Eiffel Tower out of old plastic yoghourt cartons or sticking beermats on to the garage wall – the important thing is that you do something you can take a pride in. Do something you can become good at.

4. If you have no job at all and very little money for starting up on your own, then you may still be able to abolish your boredom by establishing a small low-cost business. Window cleaning, grass cutting, gardening, cleaning other people's houses, and catering for special events are just a few of the obvious ways to begin a business venture with relatively little capital. No one with a new business to nurture can feel bored for long.

5. Improved life expectancies mean that when you retire you will probably have ten, twenty or even thirty years of life to look forward to. If you begin your retirement with no plans, no hopes, no aspirations and no expectations then you will quickly become bored. You must begin to plan your retirement years before you finish work – perhaps even planning to take on a part-time job for a year or two after formally finishing work. If you have a good pension and money isn't going to be a problem then investigate voluntary groups who might be glad of your services. And take a close look at your hobbies – will you be able to enjoy spending longer on them? Or will you need new hobbies and new interests if you are to get the best out of your retirement years?

Coping with vanity

1. If you suffer a good deal from feelings of mental or physical inadequacy then you should make a list of all your physical and mental attributes. Simply write down all your good points. Whether you are tall or small, stocky or skinny there will be good points you can be proud of. Even if you are genuinely overweight, remember that some of the most attractive people in history have been plump. Rubens never painted any skinny girls and few of the women pictured in *Playboy* magazine are thin enough to work as fashion models. Think of the mental skills and expertise you have, and write an advertisement extolling your own virtues. Think of that list – and those virtues – next time you are feeling particularly low and inferior.

85

2. If you worry unduly about your appearance and are constantly tempted to spend more than you can afford on clothes, hairdressers and so on try and see yourself as you see others.

Do you really despise everyone who has a darn in a jumper, or shun people who wear last year's fashions? Of course you don't. So why should others despise you for those very same faults?

The truth is that your idea of what other people expect is coloured not by reality but by advertisements. When you feel that you must get rid of your old suit and buy a new one simply because the cut is slightly dated you are responding to pressures deliberately exerted by commercial organisations anxious to part you from your money. Your vanity is inspired not by commonsense but by false fears inspired by skilful copywriters.

3. If you feel ashamed about your ignorance in some special area then there is one very easy remedy – do a little homework.

If you are ashamed of the fact that you don't know anything about classical music then decide to teach yourself all you need to know. If you feel that you ought to know more about international politics then start reading the newspapers and the weekly news magazines with a little more care.

Once you are confident that your areas of ignorance have been reduced you won't feel so frightened about your pride being punctured.

4. Try and encourage others to accept you for what you are. And don't take yourself too seriously. If you don't understand a joke then say so. If you find yourself at a party wearing the same outfit as another guest then try and see the funny side of it – and use the opportunity to make a new friend. Do away with your vanity and you will have much more fun. You will probably find that people will respect and admire your honesty too.

Coping with frustration

1. Try to cut down the number of people on whom you are dependent. And try to cut down the number of times you have to call in the experts. Do this and you will save yourself a lot of frustrating waiting.

Learn a little about home nursing and first aid. Learn how to repair small pieces of electrical equipment. Learn a little about basic plumbing so that you can deal with dripping taps and burst pipes. Find out how to deal with minor motor car problems – most breakdowns are caused by relatively small disorders which can be dealt with by relatively unskilled amateurs.

2. Don't be frightened to let yourself go if you feel the frustration building up inside you. If you feel rage and anger beginning to take over, and you really want to scream and shout, then go somewhere fairly quiet and private and do just that. Better still, keep a supply of really old plates somewhere so that you can smash one or two when you are feeling grumpy. Or buy a punchbag. Or a spade and enough garden to dig. Or a carpet beater. Or take up a game that involves a lot of exhausting physical work.

3. Be prepared to complain if you buy something that doesn't satisfy you. Don't just feel that you have to accept what you have been given because you don't like making a scene. Be prepared to make yourself heard – and if you have bought something that has disappointed you then don't let the shop assistant fob you off with promises to send it back to the manufacturer. It is their responsibility, not the manufacturers'. Ask for a replacement or a refund.

4. When you are planning something fairly complicated (like a house move) make a list of all the things that have got to be done. And then go through your list looking for all the places where things can go wrong. Try to make sure that you cope with most of these potential problems before they happen. Don't make plans that can be ruined if one individual lets you down. If someone really is indispensable to your plans then make sure that you allow a little extra time for them to goof up. And then remind him of what he has got to do several times before the event.

Life is undeniably and unavoidably complicated. List-making can take away a lot of the agony and leave you time and freedom to enjoy more of the ecstasy.

5. Don't allow yourself to be caught short next time there is a crisis or a strike. Keep an emergency stock of candles

87

somewhere. Have a supplementary source of heating available. If you rely on electric heating try to make sure that you have a gas cooker. And if you have a gas central-heating system then have an electric cooker. That way you will be able to cope relatively successfully if either system breaks down.

If it looks as though there may be a food strike of some kind then plan early – stock up in advance with essentials so that you won't be left completely without. Buy your petrol at one garage and get yourself known there as a regular customer. That way you are likely to get precedence next time there is a petrol strike.

Coping with ambition

1. Try to decide precisely what your ambitions are – and try to decide which parts of your life need to be taken very seriously and which parts are not quite so important. Don't let your ambition spill over into all your activities or you will soon burn yourself out.

   So, for example, if you take your job very seriously then try to relax when you are playing games. You can't be the best computer salesman in the country and the best golfer. Choose between activities which need to be taken seriously and activities which can be followed mainly for fun.

2. Don't let other people manipulate your ambitions for you. If you do then you'll probably find yourself struggling to satisfy hopes and aspirations which are impossible to fulfil. Ambition is, or should be, a very personal thing. Only you know exactly what you want out of life and how you can achieve your aims. If you spend your life struggling to satisfy someone else's ambitions then you will probably fail.

3. Remember that you can't work all the time. However great your ambitions may be and however hot that fire burning inside you may become, you will still need to relax occasionally. If you don't relax then you will get stale and ineffective. Be prepared to take time off and allow yourself to forget your problems and your worries.

   Anyone who is self-employed should have at least half a day a week put aside for something that has nothing to do with normal work. That half day should be sacrosanct. It should be wasted and frittered away on some entirely useless pastime.

4. Try to decide what you want from life – and get your priorities in some sort of order. Fame? Money? Respect? Family happiness? Academic success? You will have to be honest with yourself. If you try to satisfy contradictory ambitions then you may easily find yourself falling (painfully) between two stools. Ambitions will sometimes clash with one another and unless you have your priorities clear in your own mind you may find yourself struggling to decide which ambition to give precedence.

5. Learn to tell when you have pushed yourself too hard. There will be times in any ambitious person's life when the pressure will begin to have an adverse effect. Everyone responds to pressure and stress in a slightly different way so learn to tell just how you respond. So, for example, it may be that you will get indigestion, chest pains or wheezing when you have pushed yourself too hard. Whatever the symptom, it is a sign that you need to pull back for a while. Take things easy and perhaps even have a week or two of rest.

6. You must be able to relax – both mentally and physically – if you have powerful ambitions. You must spend some time learning how to relax effectively and efficiently so that when you are next under pressure you will be able to recharge your batteries at will. It is no good trying to learn how to relax when the pressure is on – it will be too late then.

Coping with fear

1. You must identify, recognise and face your fears. The spectre in the dark is far more dangerous than the fear you can dissect, examine and study at leisure. So decide precisely what worries you. Write down a list of your fears.

2. Whatever it is that frightens you – learn as much as you can about it. If you are frightened of aeroplanes and flying, then read books on aeroplanes and flying. If you are frightened of thunder then find out everything you can about thunder. If you are frightened of spiders then read books on spiders. Fears are often based on myths, superstitions and

half-heard facts. Learn more about the subject that gives birth to your nightmares and you might well find that your fears disappear.

3. Become a little sceptical when you hear experts telling you what is good for you, what is bad for you and what is going to happen to the world. If you listen to everything you hear and you believe everything you read then you will worry yourself into an early grave. Never heed prophets of doom and gloom until you have listened to the arguments put forward by the opposition. Read a few history books and you will soon discover that things rarely progress according to the carefully designed plans of politicians, economists or philosophers. Life always has a surprise or two for them, just where and when they least expect it.

4. If you spend a lot of time worrying about your health then make a list of all the specific fears you have – and then look at your list to see which of your fears you can do something about.

   So, for example, if you have written down heart disease and cancer on your list you can reduce your risk of suffering from either problem by watching your diet, your lifestyle, and your smoking habits. Identify all the known factors associated with your fears and then decide whether you prefer to change your life and reduce your fears or leave your life as it is and put up with your fears.

   You won't make your fears magically disappear this way but you will put them into perspective.

5. If you have a specific fear about your health then seek professional advice without delay. The woman who thinks she might have a lump in her breast and who then worries about the possibility that it could be an early cancerous growth will suffer enormously from her fears. The man who thinks his chest pains could signal a heart condition will die a thousand deaths as he waits for the massive coronary to interrupt his life.

   Both individuals would suffer far less if they sought help straight away. (And, incidentally, an early consultation will increase the chance of the doctors being able to deal with the problem quickly, effectively and permanently.)

6. When you hear something that frightens you always find out as much as you can about the source of that information.

90

Commercial organisations frequently attempt to sell their products by making people afraid. So ask yourself whether someone is deliberately trying to fill you with fear so that they can make money out of you.

Coping with lust

1. Don't let other people's claims, expectations, desires and reported sexual activities rule your own sex life. Do what comes naturally, when the time is right, with people with whom you feel comfortable. If you persistently struggle to match the alleged social norm you'll suffer agonies of doubt, suspicion, fear and inadequacy.
2. Remember that anything that is natural and comfortable is acceptable – as long as it is natural and comfortable for all the participants.
3. Don't let commercial groups or organisations push you into buying equipment, aids, clothes or other items which make you feel embarrassed, shy or in any other way uncomfortable.
   Some people drive sports cars, some drive family saloons, some prefer station wagons, and some have luxury limousines. No one car is necessarily better than all the others. They are different – that's all. The same is true for sex. Some people follow a racy, fast sex life. Others prefer a comfortable, stable, steady relationship. There isn't anything wrong with either of these alternatives. But you should choose the sex life you prefer – and not the sex life that you *think* you should prefer.
4. If sex plays a relatively minor and unimportant role in your life then refuse to feel guilty or second-rate in any way when you are faced with stories and rumours about people thinking of nothing else but sex. Different individuals have different sex drives and for many individuals complete abstinence or total celibacy is an acceptable way of life.
5. If you find yourself watching a television programme that you find sexually offensive then switch it off. If you are offered a book or magazine that you consider unacceptably porno-graphic then refuse it. If you are invited to watch a film that threatens to offer raw sexuality of a kind you find distasteful then quietly reject the invitation.

If, on the other hand, you enjoy watching raunchy TV programmes, you enjoy reading pornographic literature, or you like watching sexy films, then read and watch to your heart's content.

Whatever your personal tastes may be you are entitled to enjoy the freedom to exercise those tastes quietly and privately.

6. If you find yourself persistently tortured by desperate sexual urges which exceed your opportunities for sexual experience then you should perhaps consider reorganising your life in order to fit in with your sexual fantasies. If you continue to repress your sexual desires then you may well make yourself ill. It isn't always possible to contain a powerful sexual drive and as long as your fantasies are not dangerous, offensive or illegal you should perhaps consider allowing them to turn into reality.

Recognise your early-warning signs

Most of us have a weak point. When the pressure is getting too much we develop a physical or mental symptom that should act as a 'trigger' sign, telling us that we're doing too much, that we need to pull back a little or relax a little more.

These early-warning signs show that you are beginning to suffer real damage as a result of the stress to which you are exposed. Your stress threshold has been breached and if you don't take some fairly rapid action then your problems will merely increase.

Any physical or mental sign or symptom that becomes more apparent when you've been under pressure is an early-warning sign. But as a guide, look through the following list – it includes some of the commonest physical and mental warning signs.

Headache
Skin rash
Indigestion
Wheezing
Palpitations
Chest pains
Diarrhoea
Insomnia

Tiredness
Over-reacting to little things
Impulsive behaviour
An inability to finish tasks which have been started
Emotional responses which are difficult to control – e.g. crying
   a lot
A poor memory
An inability to concentrate
An inability to relax properly
Intolerance of noise or other stimuli
Irritability or short temper
A reduction in will-power

Whether or not it is on this list once you have spotted your early-warning sign you must learn to look out for it. When it becomes clear that your early-warning sign has been triggered then you must take some action – you need to **relax**, to pull back a little, to take some time out, and to give yourself a chance to recover. I suggest that one of the best ways to deal with the development of an early-warning sign is to use the daydreaming technique described on page 98.

Learn to cope with anxiety or panic attacks

Occasionally anxiety seems to get out of control. If you have ever had a panic attack then you will know that the name is very apt. It describes exactly what happens.

The precise symptoms vary – butterflies in the stomach, palpitations, headache, shakiness, dry mouth and an inability to concentrate on anything are some of the commonest. But though the symptoms vary the simplest, quickest and most effective way to control them is to try breathing as slowly and as deeply as you possibly can.

Take a really big breath in. Then hold it for as long as possible. Let it out. Then take another enormous breath. And hold that for as long as possible. Do this for a few minutes and you will slow down your body – and get those panic symptoms under control.

Everything you need to know about getting to sleep

Look down the list of questions on the left-hand side of this page. Every time you answer 'yes' to a question then read the appropriate notes on the right-hand side of the page.

Are you currently taking a benzodiazepine of any kind?

The benzodiazepines can disturb your sleep pattern. Even a benzodiazepine taken to help you sleep may end up by keeping you awake.

Have you recently stopped taking a benzodiazepine?

The adverse effect of benzodiazepines on sleeping patterns can last for several weeks – the exact length of time that the effect lasts will depend on the length of time for which you took the drug.

Are you kept awake by pain?

Then you must attempt to treat the cause of your pain. Or, at least, deal with the pain. Discuss your problem with your doctor. If he is unable to offer a firm diagnosis or provide you with the help you need then ask for a second opinion.

Are you kept awake by any other symptoms? e.g. breathlessness, cramp, restless legs etc.

Then you must visit your doctor for help and advice. If he is unable to offer a firm diagnosis or provide you with the help you need, then ask for a second opinion.

Are you depressed?

Then you should see your doctor for help and advice. When depression and sleeplessness go together it is the depression that needs treating.

Do you have difficulty in getting to sleep because you are too hot, too cold or in some other way uncomfortable?

Then make whatever adjustments you can to your sleeping conditions.

94

Do you have to get up at night to pass urine?	Avoid alcohol, tea, coffee and other drinks during the evening. Empty your bladder before retiring. If the problem still persists then see your doctor for a proper diagnosis and for treatment.
Are you kept awake by noise?	Try simple soundproofing – bookshelves provide an excellent sound barrier. Double glazing may help. If that fails then try wearing ear plugs.
Do you usually take a nap in the afternoon?	Then **your inability to sleep at night may** simply be a result of the fact that you don't need as much sleep as you are trying to get. Cut out the afternoon nap, or go to **bed** later.
Do you still feel alert and full of life when you go to bed?	Then you need to tire yourself out more. Any sort of exercise will do. A good brisk **walk. Or, if you can find a willing partner,** something more intimate.
Do you get kept awake by hunger?	Then have a bite of supper. Don't have anything spicy, hot or rich. A glass of milk and a couple of biscuits should do.
Are you kept awake worry about specific problems?	Keep a notebook and pencil by your bed. Write down any problems that occur to you in bed. And promise yourself that you will attend to them first thing in the morning.
Are you currently trying to lose weight?	People who are slimming seem to get less sleep than usual; their low blood sugar seems to keep them awake.
Do you worry because you don't seem to sleep as long as other people you know?	Some people need nine hours sleep a night. Others need five hours. We are all different. There is no perfect figure.

Do you worry because you don't sleep for as long as you used to?	We all need less sleep as we get older.
Do you have difficulty in making yourself comfortable at night?	Perhaps you ought to buy a new bed. Try out a few beds before you buy one. Look for one that feels right.
Do you lie awake thinking about the day's problems? Does your mind race and refuse to settle down?	Then you need to relax before you go to bed. Take a walk, soak in a hot bath, read a good book. Don't work right up to the last minute.
Do you take any prescribed drugs (apart from benzodiazepines)?	Some pills may keep you awake. Have a word with your doctor.

If you have answered all these questions and still can't explain your sleeplessness, then try a warm, milky drink before you go to bed. Or, as an occasional aid only, try a small glass of alcohol.

Relax your body

As I explained earlier in this book (on pages 7–8), fear, anxiety and stress all produce tense muscles. And when muscles become tense they tend to become sore and painful. Headaches, backache, breathing problems and a whole host of other seemingly straightforward physical problems are produced by muscles which have been tensed by stress and anxiety.

Learn to relax your muscles deliberately and you will not only avoid those physical problems but you will also get rid of some of your anxiety. Relax your muscles and you'll break the circle of tension-spasm-tension that can otherwise produce such immense difficulties.

In order to relax your muscles you must first learn just how your muscles feel when they are tight and tense. Clench your fist and you'll feel the muscles of your hand and forearm tighten and firm. Now let your fist unfold and you will feel the muscles relax. To relax properly all you have to do is stiffen and then relax the muscles of your body, group by group.

When you first start learning to relax you should choose a quiet, private place where you are not likely to be interrupted and where stimuli are least disturbing. It is difficult to begin relaxing in a busy, crowded office or bus although you will be able to do just that eventually.

Start by lying down in a darkened room where you are likely to be left alone for at least a time. You should allow a quarter of an hour for each session to start with, and you'll need to plan on spending that much time each day for a week until you have mastered the art of physical relaxation. (You will not have to relax step by step as you become more experienced, you will learn how to relax your entire body more or less instantly.) You will begin to feel better after just one session of physical relaxation; you will feel calmer and more relaxed, and your body will feel fresher and more alert.

Here is the step-by-step programme for physical relaxation:

1. Clench your left hand as firmly as you can, making a fist with your fingers. Do it well and you will see your knuckles turn white. If you now let your fist unfold you will feel the muscles relax.
2. Bend your left arm and try to make your left biceps muscle stand out as much as you can. Then relax and let the muscles ease. Let your arm lie loosely by your side, and then ignore it.
3. Relax your right hand in the same way.
4. Relax your right biceps muscles in the same way.
5. Tighten the muscles in your left foot. Curl your toes. When the foot feels as tense as you can make it let it relax.
6. Tense the muscles in your left calf. Bend the foot on that side back at the ankle to help tighten the muscles. Then let the muscles relax.
7. Straighten your leg and push your foot away from you. You should feel the muscles on the front of your thigh tighten up.
8. Relax your right foot.
9. Relax your right lower leg.
10. Relax your right thigh.

11. Lift yourself up by tightening your buttock muscles. Then let the muscles relax.
12. Contract your abdominal wall muscles. Make your waist as small as you can. And then as large as you can.
13. Tighten your chest muscles. Take a big deep breath and hold it for as long as you can. Then relax.
14. Push your shoulders back as far as they will go, then push them forwards. Shrug them up towards your ears. Then relax.
15. Tighten up the muscles in your back. Make yourself as tall as you can. Relax.
16. Pull on the muscles in your neck by moving your head first one way and then the other way. Get all the muscles tight in turn – and relax them in turn too.
17. Screw your eyes up tightly. Keep them tight. Then relax them.
18. Pull your eyebrows down. Then allow them to go as high as you can.
19. Wrinkle your nose, grit your teeth, smile broadly. Then relax those muscles in turn.
20. Push your tongue out as far as it will go. Then relax it.

While you are doing all these exercises you should take deep, regular breaths. Breathe as slowly and as deeply as you can.

Relax your mind

You can counteract the effect of stress and pressure on your body by learning to relax your mind. I think this is probably one of the easiest and most effective ways of dealing with stress and pressure. Under normal circumstances an almost unending stream of facts and feeling pour into your brain. Your eyes, ears, senses of smell and touch are all constantly gathering fresh items of information and these pieces of information are themselves producing an equally endless number of assessments and interpretations. Even when you aren't conscious of your body and mind being busy with new information, thousands of bits and pieces of information will keep you moving and adapting to your changing environment.

If you can cut the amount of information that your mind is

receiving then you will cut the number of mental responses. Researchers around the world have shown that mental relaxation can help in a number of very positive ways. There is, for example, evidence that sufferers from heart disease, high blood pressure, digestive problems and all sorts of other stress-induced troubles can benefit enormously from learning how to relax their minds.

Unfortunately, many people equate mental relaxation with meditation, and although I have nothing against meditation itself I do feel that this proves to be something of a deterrent for thousands who would benefit. I say this for two main reasons. First, the religious and semi-religious organisations which seem to be an essential part of many forms of meditation are rather frightening and disturbing to many people. Meditation has for too long been associated with shaven heads, weird clothes, pop singers and mysterious Indian gurus. Second, many of those who teach formal, traditional meditation claim that it is necessary to empty the mind completely in order to benefit. And that just isn't very easy at all. Very many people find the prospect of emptying their minds completely so daunting that they never even try.

The truth is, however, that you can enjoy all the benefits of mental relaxation without meditating, without joining any religious organisation, without going into a trance and without adopting any impossible or uncomfortable positions.

All you have to do in order to cut the flow of potentially harmful data which normally pours into your brain is to learn how to daydream. Or, to be more accurate, to revise your views on daydreaming. Most of us acquire the habit of daydreaming when we are small only to be taught by our parents and schoolteachers that it is an undesirable habit and one that we must break.

Daydreaming isn't a bad habit. It is a natural process and one which effectively helps us to relax and escape from the world's pressures. Daydreaming is a completely natural 'cut-out' process which our brains have created for their own protection. All you have to do is re-learn how to take advantage of it.

The only important thing you have to remember when you are daydreaming your cares away is that your daydream must be believable and as real as possible. You have to convince yourself (and your body) that your daydream is real. Do that and your body will respond not to the reality of the world you are living in but to the imagined world that you have created. When the film *Lawrence of Arabia* was first shown in the cinemas a few years ago cinema managers around the world were astonished to find that the sales of cold drinks and ice creams rocketed. What they didn't realise at the time was that the cinema patrons were responding not to the temperature in the cinemas but to the desert scenes they were watching on the screen. The people watching the film were so taken with what they saw that their bodies responded as though the desert was real. It didn't matter if it was freezing in the cinema – the patrons still wanted to buy ice creams to cool themselves down.

You can use exactly the same principles to help you cope with life's stresses and strains. To start with you'll probably need to begin your daydreaming somewhere quiet and peaceful where you can cut out the world fairly easily. Later on, when you've mastered the art of daydreaming, you'll be able to do it just about anywhere.

Lie yourself down on your bed, close the door, take the telephone off the hook and draw the curtains. Put a 'Do Not Disturb' notice on the door if you can find one.

Now, try to think of some scene from the past, some scene that you found relaxing and peaceful. Try a beach scene from a happy holiday memory, for example. With your eyes closed take big deep breaths as slowly as you possibly can and try to feel the warmth of the sun on your face. Don't let anyone else into your daydream, by the way. If you let people come in then you'll either end up with a fantasy (which won't be restful at all) or else you'll end up chatting or, worse still, arguing with them.

Just imagine that you are lying by yourself on a deserted beach. Imagine that you can hear the sound of the waves breaking on the shore some way away. And try to feel the warm, soft sand underneath you. Smell the salty air and the light perfume of your favourite sun oil. Hear the seagulls circling high overhead and allow a gentle breeze to play over your body. Keep the action quiet and peaceful but just flood your mind with all these images of a happy memory.

Once your mind has been convinced your body will be convinced too. The accumulated pressures and stresses of the real world will disappear as your body takes it easy. You can gain just as much from your daydream as you ever could hope to gain from spending real time down there on the beach. As your mind is filled with these peaceful thoughts so your body will begin to respond. Your blood pressure will fall, your muscles will become relaxed, your stomach will stop pumping out acid and your whole body will benefit.

You don't have to restrict yourself to this one particular daydream, of course. You can build a library of your very own private daydreams. You can store up a valuable collection of happy memories designed to enable you to escape from the realities of the world. Perhaps you had a happy day in the country, sitting by a small stream and watching leaves and sticks floating down in the water. Perhaps you had a beautifully relaxing day on a mountainside. It doesn't matter what memories you use for your daydreaming as long as they were happy and peaceful. Indeed, you can create false daydreams if you like just as long as you make them really convincing. Use scenes from films or television programmes if you like. If your mind believes that you are there then your body will believe too, and will respond accordingly.

Daydreaming has one enormous advantage over meditation. Instead of having to empty your mind completely and replace real anxieties with a clinically clean, empty space, you will be replacing your natural fears with loving, comfortable memories which will themselves have a useful and positive effect. When you empty your head of damaging stressful thoughts and fill it with nothingness then you halt the damage caused by the pressures of the outside world. But when you empty your head of damaging thoughts and fill it with joyful memories you don't just halt the damage, you do much, much more. You can build up your inner strength. Negative emotions, such as fear and anxiety, can do a great deal of harm. But positive emotions, such as happiness, can contribute enormously to your all-round health. Daydreaming is good for you.

Take a break

One of the simplest ways in which to avoid stress is to change your way of life temporarily. So, when you are feeling tired, fed up or exhausted, or your early-warning signs are appearing with increasing frequency, consider taking a day or two away from your problems. Just go away somewhere for a change of air or scenery.

Unhappily, many people spend their valuable holiday period struggling to accumulate a new series of exotic experiences and

101

photographs with which to entertain and impress the neighbours at home. Such a holiday is merely likely to contribute to your annual stress overdraft rather than to help in any way to diminish it. Amazingly there are now many ways of making sure that your holiday period ends up producing more stress – rather than helping you reduce your levels of stress. So, for example, a growing number of people are buying mobile homes and touring wild countryside miles away from normal, everyday problems. Or they are buying tumbledown cottages where there are no telephones. The psychological value of having such a retreat can be enormous but so many people spoil the effect by attempting to improve the market value of their escape by introducing all the services and facilities they originally went there to escape. There isn't any point in buying a caravan to escape from the real world if you then spend all your time tinkering with the fridge, the TV set and the portable microwave oven.

So, if you are planning a break because you need a rest from stress and pressure, make sure that you don't make this sort of mistake. Do something that will allow you to unwind – perhaps take a few days by the seaside or in the countryside where you can dress informally, stay in bed until you feel like getting up, go to bed when you're tired and potter around according to the way you feel rather than according to the way you think you ought to behave.

If you've got children and you need to get away from them for a day or two, then ask relatives or friends for help. There may be another couple who would happily have your children for a couple of days in return for a similar favour at some future date.

Remember the values of organisation

If a builder tried to erect a cathedral without any plans he would undoubtedly end up in trouble. On a less dramatic scale it is equally true that people who do not plan ahead often end up in a terrible mess – when with a little forward planning they would have been able to avoid many problems.

The housewife who makes a shopping list and then ensures that she buys everything she needs on a single visit to the supermarket will have fewer domestic crises than the housewife who buys purely on impulse. The motorist who remembers to have his car serviced and keep the tank and radiators, etc. filled will have fewer unexpected breakdowns than the motorist who leaves things to chance. The student who plans his workload and decides how much time needs to be allotted to each individual project will be far less likely to end up with a half completed workload.

Bad organisation and a failure to plan ahead will often lead to anxiety, to crises, to increased stress loads – and to a need for tranquillisers.

To organise your life efficiently and effectively follow this advice:

1. Keep a notebook and pencil by you at all times. Write down any problems that seem significant or any things that you have to remember. Diaries really aren't much good because there is never enough room. You can throw away notebooks when they are filled much easier than you can change diaries. There are several benefits to be gained from using notebooks. You'll not have to spend hours wondering what it was that you were so anxious to remember for one thing! More important, when it's down on paper, many a problem seems far less significant. Leave it and come back to it and what seemed insuperable may have sorted itself out.

2. Keep a diary and get into the habit of examining it each morning to make sure that you know just what you have to do. Put a note in your diary about a week ahead of all birthdays, anniversaries and events that need advance planning. That way you should have time to plan purchases, cards and so on.

3. When you've got a really difficult problem to solve write down all the alternative solutions in your notebook. Keep the list somewhere and add new solutions as they occur to you. Keep it by your bedside because good ideas often pop into your head last thing at night just when you're about to go to sleep. Then when you need to make a decision look down your list and select the best possible solution. You'll probably find that by this time one particular answer stands out.

4. Keep a filing system to enable you to store bills, receipts and important letters where you can find them. If you just stuff documents into drawers and pockets then you'll waste hours later. If you don't want to buy a filing cabinet then use old

brown envelopes, just writing on the outside what they contain within.

5.   When you are planning some special event – such as a move or large celebration – then keep a special master-plan to help you keep things running smoothly. List everything that needs to be done and mark off the dates by which each problem has to be solved. You can cut your worry and anxiety enormously by doing this.

The escape clause

There is one final way to deal with stress that is getting unbearable. One way that will work even if you can't take a break or a holiday. A way that will enable you to avoid problems and pressures even when you can't officially get away.

Take to your bed.

Charles Darwin used to become ill to give himself an excuse to rest in bed for a while. So did Florence Nightingale, Marcel Proust, Sigmund Freud and many, many other famous and successful people.

Don't, however, make the mistake of taking to your bed with 'tiredness', 'anxiety', 'stress' or 'tension' as your problem. You'll be encouraged (or forced) to carry on. And you'll probably end up with genuine, physical symptoms produced by too much stress.

Instead, produce some mild physical symptoms for just long enough to get you a break away from the pressure and stress of the real world. A little muscular backache, a mild bout of flu, a bad headache – all will usually earn you a day or two's respite. Somehow a bad back seems far more acceptable to most employers than 'mental exhaustion' or 'stress'.

Remember, this is a last resort, of course. I don't want to encourage you to become a malingerer. But using the escape clause is far preferable to taking a benzodiazepine.

Remember that depression and anxiety can be contagious

It has always seemed to me that one of the silliest things that psychiatrists do (and to be honest, they do quite a lot of silly things) is to put all their depressed and anxious patients into the same wards. Nothing could be better designed to exacerbate existing problems. When you are feeling miserable and depressed the last thing you want is to be dumped in a room with a couple of dozen other people who feel just as low as you do. When you're feeling tense and anxious, mixing with a host of other tense and anxious people will simply make you feel worse. Depression and anxiety may not be infectious in the strictest sense of the word but they are contagious in that we can all of us be influenced by the moods and feelings of others; if you're the sort of person who tends to suffer from anxiety a good deal then mixing with anxious people will undoubtedly make your problem much worse.

Obviously, therefore, you should try as much as you can to avoid spending too much time in the company of people who are constantly suffering with their nerves. If, on looking around, you see nothing but blank faces, frowns and scowls, gloomy eyes and tear-stained cheeks, then perhaps you should try to make some new and more cheerful friends.

And perhaps you ought to let yourself go a little occasionally. These are very serious times and there are lots of things that do need attention. But if you let all your problems fill your mind constantly you'll be far less able to deal with them. So, while you're looking for brighter and jollier friends perhaps you could help yourself a little by buying yourself a toy or a comic, by buying some balloons, by playing games on the paving slabs, by buying some bubbles or whatever else you fancy. The sillier the escapade, and the more you enjoy it, the more good it will do you.

Rock away the blues

A child who is very upset and troubled will often sit hunched up and rock backwards and forwards very gently. A mother whose baby is crying will pick up the infant, put it in her arms and cradle it backwards and forwards. Child and mother do this quite naturally, without any teaching or prompting, because the rocking motion helps to relax and body and drain away accumulated tensions. No one really knows just how this works, but it seems likely that the rhythmic motion aids in counteracting urgent messages which are being sent from the muscles to the brain. The anxiety and tension

105

tightens up muscles but the rocking motion loosens them again.

You can use these same principles to help you deal with stress by buying yourself a rocking chair. Sit and rock yourself backwards and forwards, just as Grandma used to do, and you'll gradually soothe yourself and send away the accumulated troubles and tensions of the day.

The rocking chair is a wooden Valium. But it has no side effects and no uncontrollable addictive properties.

Let your emotions show

Most of us are taught to hide our emotions whenever possible. We are taught to keep our anger deep inside us when we're cross, to refuse to allow anyone to see us cry, to hide our pride and so on. As a nation the British are particularly prone to suppressing their emotions in this way – and men and boys are far more likely to be taught the importance of emotional suppression than girls or women. The truth is, however, that it is much, much safer to let emotions out than it is to bottle them up inside you.

Take crying for example. Because crying is such an obvious physical manifestation of distress many people grow up to regard it as a sign of weakness and emotional instability. Boys in particular are taught that it is unforgivable to cry in public, and that they should always bottle up their feelings.

Bottling up tears can produce all sorts of problems. It can certainly result in mental and physical symptoms of anxiety and distress developing. There is now even evidence to show that tears that are produced by emotional distress contain special substances that the body needs to get rid of. Keep those tears inside you and you keep the unwanted chemicals too – and that could be dangerous. Crying is a natural response designed to rid the body of unnecessary substances and to attract attention from those around us.

Just as crying is sometimes good for you so it is also sometimes wise to let your anger out. Your body is designed for physical action. When things go wrong or you are threatened in anyway your body will automatically prepare itself for physical activity. Your muscles will tighten, your blood pressure will go up and your whole body will be made ready. These preparations are physiologically quite sound, of course. If you're trying to get out of a burning house or cope with a burglar then you need every ounce of muscle power you can lay your hands on.

Unfortunately, these days physical preparations for stressful situations tend to be rather useless. Your body will be prepared for action that won't come and your muscles will be tensed quite unnecessarily. When you're facing a stubborn clerk, a difficult traffic warden or a frustrating shop assistant, then physical action will be inappropriate if not illegal. All this does, however, explain why, when you're frustrated or thwarted, you may well feel like punching someone, breaking a window, screaming or smashing some china. Your body wants you to do something physical but the problems you are most likely to find yourself facing won't be the sort that can be solved with physical activity.

In these circumstances you would be wise to adapt your behaviour a little to fit in with your body's natural preparations. I'm not suggesting that you should start hitting people who annoy you or throwing things at anyone who offends you at all. But there are lots of simple, practical ways in which you can get rid of these developed aggressions. Remember, if you don't get rid of these aggressive feelings then they'll just get stored up inside you and will probably produce problems in the future.

You can, if you wish, get rid of your excess energy by taking part in some hectic or even violent sporting activity. Hitting a squash or tennis ball or kicking a football can be a pretty good way to get rid of aggressive feelings for example. Or you can paint the face of someone you hate on to a punchball and try hitting the hell out of that. Or buy one of those games where you hit a ball which is attached by a long piece of elastic to a solid base – and hit that as hard as you can when you are feeling particularly aggressive. Or simply try taking a pile of old plates into the garage or down the garden and smashing them one by one!

Whatever it is you choose, getting rid of those aggressive feelings will leave you far healthier than if you let them store up inside you.

CASE HISTORIES

Over the years I have seen and spoken to hundreds of tranquilliser users. I've included these case histories because patients can often learn as much from other sufferers as they can from experts.

I have, of course, changed the names to protect the innocent (and the guilty).

Mrs T.F.

Right up until the time when the last of them left home for good I honestly thought that I'd enjoy having a bit of time to myself. When you've always had children to look after and worry about everything seems a bit flat without them, however. On the Sunday morning after our Doreen got married and went to live with Tony in their new flat I remember feeling terribly lonely. It was as though my life had suddenly ended.

Don't get me wrong, I've always loved my husband and he's always been very good to me. But my life had always revolved around the children. George had his darts, his fishing and his job. And he had all his mates too. I just had the children and they were my whole life. When they'd gone I felt as though my life had come to an end. I just didn't have anything left to do. George hasn't had any meals at home for years now. He has his Sunday lunch, of course, but the rest of the time he either eats in the canteen or in the pub. Or else he makes himself some sandwiches. He didn't really need me. Not in the way that the children needed me.

My periods stopped at about the same time too. My fifty-first birthday was one of the most miserable days of my life. Doreen had got married about a fortnight before. And the doctor had told me that I'd started on the change that week. I'd been to see him because I hadn't seen a period for nearly a year. George forgot my birthday again – he hardly ever remembers. And when he'd gone out to work that morning I just sat down on the bed and cried and cried and cried. I sobbed my heart out that day.

I remember thinking that there just wasn't much point to living any more. The children didn't need me. And George didn't need me. I didn't have anything to do. I'd spent all my life being useful to other people and I just didn't know what else to do.

Well, I spent about a week sitting in the living room staring at the walls and I can tell you that several times I thought how much I'd have liked to have died. Not that I'd have ever done anything about it, of course. I wouldn't have tried to do anything silly. I wouldn't know how to set about it. And it wouldn't be fair, would it?

I don't think that George ever knew how I felt. I always tried to put on a brave face for him. I didn't want to worry him. He wasn't

111

all that happy at work at the time – they were having some dispute and he was worried about his job. Besides we'd never really talked about things like that. Not about how we felt inside. I didn't think it would be right to burden him with my troubles.

In the end I went back to see the doctor again. I told him that I was feeling very depressed and asked him for a tonic. He told me that it was probably just my hormones, just the menopause, and he gave me some tranquillisers to help me. I asked him if they were Valium and he said they weren't. In fact I found out later that he'd been a little bit naughty there – they weren't Valium, it is true, but they were something very similar. Anyway, he gave me a prescription for a huge bottleful and told me to go back and see him in a month or so.

I took the tablets for over a year and it was without a doubt the worst, the very worst year of my life. To be perfectly honest I can't remember very much about it, it all seems a blur now, but I remember spending a lot of time crying and it all getting so bad that even George noticed that something was wrong. He was ever so good. He came to me one Saturday night when he was due to go to a darts tournament and spent ages trying to make me tell him what was wrong. When I couldn't he thought that I was keeping something secret and he got quite cross. The trouble was I couldn't tell him because I didn't know myself.

Then by accident I came across an article in a women's magazine. It was about Valium and drugs like it and there was a long list of other tablets that were supposed to have a similar effect. I noticed that the tablets I was taking were listed there. That was the first time I realised that they were tranquillisers.

The next time I went to the doctor I asked him if I could try without the tablets. He said he thought that I was being silly and that the tablets wouldn't do me any harm but told me that if I wanted to try without them I should try cutting down slowly – to give my body time to get used to being without them.

I should have listened to him, I know, but I was so desperate to stop the tablets that I just stopped them there and then. I didn't take another one at all. It was terrible.

I got the shakes, I felt sick and I couldn't stand up properly. I just didn't know what I was doing. Everything came to a head one day when I was in one of the local supermarkets doing the

112

shopping. I can't remember a thing about what happened but I found myself standing outside on the pavement with a man in a grey suit, and a couple of policemen with me. One of them might have been a policewoman. I can't remember.

They said that I'd put some baked beans in my own bag and tried to steal them. I didn't know what they were talking about and to this day I can't tell you how the beans got into my bag. Funny thing is that neither George nor I liked baked beans anyway. I never buy them. The police wouldn't listen to me, however. They took me down to the station and made George come and get me. They told us both I'd be charged.

I know it sounds funny to say it but in a way that was probably the best thing that could have happened to me. George took me along to the doctor and told him what had happened. The doctor didn't seem all that interested but George got very cross and said he wanted me to see a specialist. So the doctor fixed me up with an appointment at the hospital.

The specialist was wonderful. He wrote a letter to the court for me explaining that I'd been acting under the influence of drugs. And the magistrates just gave me a warning and dismissed the case. The specialist helped me get off the tranquillisers and he arranged for me to see a gynaecologist for some help with my menopause problems. I had some special hormone tablets that made all the difference.

People always talk about psychiatrists as though they are a bit odd but that specialist was a psychiatrist and he was really kind to me. It was as though he really understood. When I'd got off the pills he explained that I had to start rebuilding my life without the children and start living for myself for a change.

It isn't easy and I'm not pretending that I don't still have bad days. But I've joined several societies and I get out of the house quite a lot now. I'm going to evening classes twice a week to study English and French and for the first time in my life I've got ambitions of my own. I want to go to France and I've told George that even if he won't come with me I'll go anyway; by myself if necessary. I want to do a bit of writing too and I've already had an article published in the local newspaper. It made me feel very proud.

I still feel quite bitter about the doctor who gave me the

113

tranquillisers. I don't think he helped me at all.

Mrs J.G.

At the time nearly everyone I know was taking Valium or something like it. My mother and father were both taking it and so was my sister. My best friend was taking some little blue tablets that weren't Valium but were something very similar. And I know for a fact that her seven-year-old was being given half a tablet every evening to help him get to sleep.

So I wasn't really surprised when my doctor gave me a prescription for them too. I went to see him because I'd had a couple of little funny turns. I don't really know how to describe them but they weren't anything too much. I only went to the surgery because my sister said I ought to. Looking back I think that they were probably just quite normal little patches of anxiety. One was when my youngest was an hour late from school. I got myself into quite a state. I decided that he'd been run over and I rang my husband and got him to come home from work. He was furious, I remember, because he arrived home just about the same time as Jason who had been playing on the swings with some friends. The other time was when my period was ten days late. I'd missed taking a couple of my pills and I didn't dare tell my husband. I knew he didn't want any more children and he'd have gone berserk if I'd told him. So I got myself into quite a state over that too.

Anyway, as I say, my sister said I ought to tell the doctor. He listened to me for about two minutes and then handed me a prescription for some tablets. He told me to take them three times a day for a fortnight and said that if they helped I could have more without coming into the surgery but just by ringing up for a prescription to be left out for me.

I took them for months and months. I can't remember exactly how long but it was quite a time. And as the months went by I needed the tablets more and more. I started getting really bad anxiety attacks at least once every day. I'd break out in a sweat and shake and get all het up over absolutely nothing at all.

I was convinced that without the tablets I'd really be in a bad state so I gradually increased the dose I was taking. After six months I was taking twelve or fifteen tablets every day. Some days

I took even more. Amazingly I never had any difficulty in getting tablets. I just had to ring up the surgery and leave a message asking for a fresh supply to be left out. I got the prescriptions for 200 tablets at a time and I think that I could have got pills every day if I'd wanted them. Well, that's perhaps a bit of an exaggeration but not all that much.

It was a television programme I saw that eventually frightened me off the pills. I'd never thought about them being addictive or dangerous until I saw that programme. It scared the wits out of me and I rang the doctor to try and make an appointment. I wanted to ask him about them. But the earliest appointment I could get was a fortnight away. So I didn't bother. Instead I just tried stopping the pills myself. On the television programme they'd said that you had to cut the pills down slowly so that's what did. I just cut down by limiting myself to so many pills every day.

It was harder, much harder, than I'd thought it would be. I felt sick, I got really bad shakes and I used to walk around the house sobbing to myself nearly all day. But the programme had really terrified me and I was determined to stop them so I persevered.

I got myself down to six a day before I finally went to see the doctor. He said I was probably sensible to cut down and he gave me advice about how to cut out the rest. But to be perfectly honest he didn't tell me anything I hadn't already worked out for myself.

I found that the most difficult thing to cope with was the feeling of anxiety that I kept getting. It was much, much worse than the feeling I'd got when I'd first gone to the doctor's. On the television programme they had said that you could learn how to relax yourself quite easily and so I bought a paperback that was supposed to help you deal with stress and it was really quite good. I followed some exercises and found that although I still got the anxieties I didn't suffer half as much as I had to start with.

I've been off the tranquillisers for two months now and I still get some little anxiety attacks. But nothing worse than I had when I started taking the tablets. And nothing I can't cope with. I certainly feel a good deal better than I did when I was taking the pills. The irony is that taking the pills made me so bad that my original problems seem very insignificant in comparison. I certainly don't think I ever had any problems that merited treatment with powerful drugs. I think my doctor should have told me that

115

everyone gets anxiety from time to time and just taught me a little bit about relaxation. Still, he's always very busy and I suppose it's easier to hand over a prescription. That's what they're trained to do and that's what a lot of people expect anyway.

Mr A.C.

Looking back I suppose I've always been what you'd call a bit of a 'workaholic'. I think it all goes back to the days when I was a boy, under pressure to do well at school. My parents were always giving me targets and always pushing me and telling me to do better and work harder. I don't ever remember being praised for anything I did – just admonished when I didn't do as well as they expected.

When I left school and started work at the bank I just carried on in exactly the same conscientious way. I worked longer hours than any of the other trainees, did more studying at home than any other young employees and spent hours reading books and journals that were filled with obscure and erudite articles on the workings of the banking system.

That sort of devotion is rewarded, of course, and I'd only been at the bank for a few years when I was given my first real responsibility. By the time I was in my late twenties I was managing a small branch in the suburbs of London and even my parents had to admit (albeit grudgingly) that I seemed to be getting on reasonably well.

The trouble with being a workaholic is that even when you're successful you don't stop. By the time I got my first decent-sized branch to manage in my mid-thirties I had a duodenal ulcer and a mild heart condition. I'd married by then, of course, and my wife was constantly nagging me to slow down a bit and take things a little easier but I just couldn't.

I started taking Mogadon to help me sleep when I was thirty-six and about a year later I added Valium to help me relax a little during the daytime. You'd have thought that I'd have had more sense but I was still pushing myself incredibly hard, working all day at the bank and then taking work home with me in my briefcase. I was nearly always first at the bank in the morning and always last to leave at night. I was the only person in the bank to work through lunch and all tea and coffee breaks.

I'd been taking the Mogadon and the Valium for about a year when I first noticed problems developing but it was another six months before I did anything about it. The first symptom I noticed was drowsiness during the mornings – I fell asleep once or twice when customers were with me and once I actually fell asleep when my area manager was down for the day to discuss some major loans we were considering.

When my concentration started to wander and I began to forget important meetings quite regularly, I went back to my doctor to ask him for a check-up. He hadn't the time for a proper examination so he sent me along to one of those commercial medical screening centres where they spend several hours going over you with a fine toothcomb, taking X-rays, blood samples and so on.

The doctor at the screening centre seemed surprised when I told him how long I'd been on the tablets. He was quite straight with me and told me there and then that he thought they were probably responsible for the symptoms I was getting. He told me to go back to see my own doctor and ask for help in coming off them.

Coming off the pills was absolutely terrible for several months. I couldn't sleep at all, I couldn't settle down in the evening, I could hardly get through a day's work without panicking, and I started to get all sorts of strange symptoms – like sweating and really bad headaches.

My own family doctor was quite helpful. I must make that quite clear. He really did help me quite a lot. But it was my wife who helped me most of all. She was absolutely marvellous. She and my assistant at the bank.

My assistant covered for me for quite a long time, telling important callers that I was busy when I was simply incapable of taking their calls, and telling Head Office that I was out visiting clients when I was just too woozy to get out of bed and go to the bank at all. If Head Office had really known what was going on they'd have gone berserk because I had quite a lot of financial responsibility.

My wife helped in two ways. First, she was very supportive during the worst stages of giving up the tablets. She helped in a lot of practical ways, going round with me to make sure I didn't forget things I had to do, keeping aspirin tablets for the headaches and so on. She's never been able to cope very well with sickness but she was marvellous to me then.

117

But the most important thing she did was give me confidence in myself. Slowly she managed to encourage me to take things a little easier, to hold back a little and to be prepared to spend a little time away from the bank occasionally. She didn't entirely cure me of my 'workaholism', of course – I don't think that's really curable – but she enabled me to control it much more effectively.

That was vitally important because if she hadn't helped me in that way I think I'd have ended up just going back on to the tablets again. As it is now I still work too hard but at least I can switch off occasionally at nights and at weekends. I go for walks, I do a bit of gardening, and we spend some time in our caravan in the country. I've even been known to do a bit of fishing.

It took about four months altogether to get off the tablets and get back to something approaching normality. I can sleep fairly well now and I don't get panic attacks any more. And I can tell you one thing – I shan't ever take a sleeping tablet or a tranquilliser again.

Mrs O.L.

I really don't know why I let my doctor give me the tablets at all. I've been a qualified nurse for over thirty years and I've known lots of patients who have had problems with the benzodiazepines. I always swore that I'd never take them.

I went to see him after I retired because I felt low and wanted some help. I don't know what I expected him to do. When I came out of the surgery with a prescription for a tranquilliser I was half tempted to throw it away. I walked past the pharmacy twice before I finally went in and got the tablets. Even then I was tempted to throw them away. But I didn't.

Retiring early wasn't my choice. I think I'd have stayed on longer if I'd had the opportunity. But I was encouraged to take early retirement and they made it clear that they thought it would be best for everyone if I did. I don't think it was a question of my not being able to do my job properly. I think they just wanted to reduce the staffing levels and getting people to take early retirement was the easiest solution.

Trouble was that my job had been the most important part of my life for a long, long time. Ever since my husband had died, in fact. He was only thirty-eight when he died. It was a massive heart

118

attack and quite unexpected. I don't think I ever really got over the shock. We had no children and there wasn't anything else that I could lose myself in except my work.

I took the tablets for about eighteen months altogether. They did absolutely nothing for me and I can't imagine why I carried on taking them. I suppose I just started because I wanted to try something, anything that would offer some hope, and I carried on because I got hooked.

I think I'd have still been taking them today if the doctor who had prescribed them hadn't died and been replaced by a younger fellow who knew a bit more about drugs and drug problems. He got very cross when I told him how long I'd been taking the tablets and although he didn't say anything specific about it I could tell that he was critical of the other doctor's prescribing habits. I'd been getting the pills on repeat prescriptions for ages and I don't think I'd seen anyone for over six months.

He helped me stop taking the pills and asked me why I didn't start looking around for another job. I know it sounds really stupid but I hadn't even thought of finding another job. I'd just assumed that at my age I was on the scrap heap for good.

The good thing about having a qualification, of course, is that you can nearly always find something to do. And I managed to get a job working in an old people's home where they needed a part-time nursing assistant. It wasn't anywhere near as grand a job as the one I'd had before. And I didn't get paid the same rates. But I've been doing it for about three months now and I really enjoy it. I've also started work with a voluntary organisation which helps people trying to get off tranquillisers. I think it's an enormous problem that is still underestimated by the medical profession. And until more doctors understand what damage they are doing I think the problem is going to get worse.

Mrs W.M.

I remember when I was a tiny tot my mother and father once shouted at me when we were on the beach at Paignton because I ran around on the beach without my blouse on. I was four at the time but I can still remember feeling very ashamed of myself for years

119

afterwards. I felt as though I'd done something really dirty and horrible. My mother and father were both keen churchgoers and they both held very strong views about things like nudity in public.

When I was a teenager I didn't go out with boys or go to dances or things like that very much because my parents didn't approve of that sort of thing. I met Tony, my husband, at a Christmas social organised by a local anti-abortion group that my mother supported. When he gave me a goodnight kiss after our fourth date a couple of weeks later I felt really excited. It was ever such a funny feeling. Part of me felt ashamed and guilty and part of me felt quite exhilarated. I really felt as though I'd done something desperately daring.

When we married about four months later we hadn't progressed past the kissing stage. I'd have happily let him be more daring but I think he was even more terrified about the whole thing than I was. We used to sit in the cinema holding hands and I could feel him shaking and sweating. I think he was terrified that someone would see us and tell his mother and father. They were even stricter than mine.

You might have imagined that our first night in bed together would have been a complete disaster but in fact as far as I was concerned it was remarkably successful. I know a lot of women have problems enjoying sex and so on but I had an orgasm straight off. It was marvellous and I remember being quite disappointed when he couldn't do it again straight afterwards. I didn't know anything about sex or men or anything. All I knew was that I liked it and wanted to do it again.

Tony really was very shocked, I'm afraid. He didn't know much more about sex than I did but he had been taught that it was basically just for having babies. He certainly didn't think it was for enjoying and he was startled when I seemed to like it. He said it wasn't normal for a woman to enjoy sex like that and the next night when I wanted him to do it again he got very cross indeed and said he was surprised at me. I know it sounds difficult to believe but he said he wanted to wait to see if I got pregnant before he did it again.

Well, I'm afraid that as far as I was concerned that just wasn't good enough. I'd really enjoyed sex that first time and if I couldn't have him then I certainly wasn't going to completely forget about sex until the time came for us to try and make a baby again. For the first time in my life I tried masturbating. It wasn't as good as the real thing but it was still very enjoyable. I honestly hadn't ever masturbated before then. Funny, isn't it?

By the time we'd been married three months I was masturbating two or three times every day. Tony used to spend two or three nights a month away from home and I used to look forward to those nights because it meant that I could lie in bed and masturbate freely for as long as I liked. I used to cover myself in perfume, put on something silky and sexy, close my eyes and have the most extraordinary fantasies. I'd play Barry Manilow records all the time. I'd do it in the afternoons too sometimes. I'd just go up into the bedroom, draw the curtains and imagine that I was being ravished by some gorgeous Eastern potentate.

One afternoon Tony came home from work early and unexpectedly. Because of the record player I didn't hear him come in. He couldn't find me downstairs and so he just walked upstairs and came into the bedroom. When he saw me he just stood there and stared. He didn't say anything but just went very white then turned round and walked out. A few hours later his mother rang me to tell me that he wouldn't be coming back. She said some really dreadful things and called me some awful names. When I put the telephone down I was really shaking.

After that I went to the doctor several times but I just told him that I was having marital problems. I didn't dare tell him what the problems really were because I thought he'd think me disgusting. The doctor gave me something called lorazepam to take during the daytime and because I couldn't sleep at night he gave me nitrazepam for the evenings.

Although he told me to take only three of the tablets during the day I was so upset that I took twice that many. I wanted to knock myself out and the tablets certainly helped with that. Looking back what really frightens me was that he never told me that I shouldn't drive while I was taking the tablets and I must have had dozens of really narrow escapes. I hit a milk float one morning when I was going shopping and another time I drove straight into a tree.

He didn't tell me that I shouldn't drink either and because the sleeping tablets didn't really help me very much I used to have half a bottle of sherry with them. I had to cut out the past because all I could hear was Tony's mother yelling at me down the phone and all

I could see was his face when he'd burst in on me like that. I still go all funny when I think about it.

I carried on with the pills for about three or four months. The doctor was very good about letting me have them because he knew that Tony and I had split up. He just let me collect the pills from the receptionist. Well, I got a prescription from the receptionist and got the pills from the chemists.

I don't know how long it would have gone on if I hadn't had my accident but I suppose it could still have been the same now. I call it an accident because that's really what it was. I couldn't get to sleep one night and I just kept taking pills and drinking sherry to try and shut out the world. I wasn't trying to do anything silly. That's what my doctor calls it: 'doing something silly'. He means kill yourself but he doesn't like to use the words.

It was my mother who found me. I don't know how she came to be there but she says I telephoned her. I don't remember that. She called an ambulance straight away, of course, and they just took me into the hospital. They pumped me out and took me on to the ward. I can just remember that. It was horrible. Really horrible.

A psychiatrist came to see me the next morning and because I was feeling so tired and so completely drained I told him everything. I don't think I would have told him if I hadn't been feeling like that. I just told him absolutely everything. When I'd finished I expected him to get up and walk away. I thought he'd be disgusted too. I was quite surprised when he didn't say something nasty.

He stayed with me for ever such a long time. I'll always remember that. He explained that it wasn't really me who had the problem but Tony and that it was quite normal for a woman to have responded in the way I did. I can't tell you the relief I felt. I suddenly felt very calm and quite at peace. It was very odd.

I wouldn't see Tony when he came into the hospital later that day and I wouldn't see my parents either. I just didn't want to see them. It wasn't that I couldn't cope with them or anything, it was just that I didn't need their sort of sympathy. I just wanted to be left alone to sort things out for myself.

I still see the phsyciatrist and I've been reading a lot of books about human sexuality and so on since then. I still haven't seen Tony and I've only seen my parents once or twice. I haven't had

122

any pills at all since I came out of the hospital and I haven't felt the need for them. I've still got a problem, I know that, but at least I know what the problem is now. I haven't masturbated since Tony came in and found me and I don't think I could have sex with anyone just yet. But at least I'm doing something about the problem.

And I'll tell you this; if I ever have a little girl and she wants to go running around on the beach without her top on I won't stop her!

Mrs A.K.

Before I was married I used to work in Woolworths. It wasn't much of a job really but we used to have some great laughs there and the girls were a smashing bunch. I fell for Janice when Barry and I were still courting and we had to get married a bit quicker than we'd anticipated. Still, I suppose we were lucky in some ways. Because I was carrying, Barry's uncle Norman managed to get us a council flat. It was on the top floor of one of those tower blocks on the Pilkington Estate. I had to leave work, of course, but at the time it didn't worry me at all. I quite liked being a housewife and I used to always try and have something nice for Barry when he came home from work. He works out of doors most of the time and he's always got a big appetite. He likes chips mostly with everything.

We never got round to using any contraceptives after Janice. Barry never liked using those things and he didn't like the idea of me going on the pill because he said it wasn't safe. Simon and Pamela came quite quickly after Janice and although the flat soon got crowded I didn't mind too much when they were little. I was sterilised after Pamela, by the way.

Some people seem to find looking after kids tiring, but I like it. They were never much trouble when they were little and although there wasn't much room for them to play we had some good fun. Barry brought a kitten home one day. We weren't supposed to have any pets. He smuggled it in and we kept a tray with old newspapers for it up a corner. It was really **great**.

I always thought that I might go back to work when the kids were at school. When I left, the manager at the store told me that they'd always be pleased to see me back again and I wouldn't have minded going back there. Although really to be honest I always wanted to be a beautician. You know in the big stores how they have those beauty counters where the girls stand around selling perfumes, lipsticks and make-up? That must be a great job. I had a friend who knew someone who worked there and she said that they got some free make-up every week so that they'd always look good.

But the kids had all been at school for over a year, and Barry kept saying that he didn't want me to go out to work. He said his mates would think he couldn't earn enough to keep us if I was seen working, and that he didn't want me working in a shop anyway. He said he didn't want me standing around being chatted up. When I said I was fed up with being on my own in the flat all day he shouted and said why didn't I tidy the place up a bit and do a bit of decorating. He said it was a hole and it smelt of cat pee and he threatened to get rid of Tabby. That's the cat. I don't know what I'd do without Tabby to keep me company. I really don't. The thing is I suppose that I get awfully lonely and Tabby's sometimes the only person I speak to all day from when the kids go out to school to when they come back in again. I tried to keep the flat looking clean and nice but sometimes I just wanted to scream and I hated it at all.

I don't think I'd have ever gone to the doctor except for the fact that when my Mum came round with Janice's birthday present six months ago she could see that I'd been crying. She went out to the phone there and then and rang the surgery and made me an appointment. The doctor was very nice but ever so busy and I didn't really know what to tell him anyway. He asked me if I'd been depressed and I said I supposed I had a bit. He gave me a prescription for some little yellow tablets and said I had to take them three times a day and go back to him a fortnight later. I went back but that doctor wasn't there then. The doctor I saw said I should keep on with the tablets for as long as I was feeling low. He said they'd help me.

Well, I suppose they did help for a while. They stopped me worrying and made me feel a bit calmer for a week or two. But it was funny really because I slowly seemed to lose interest in things. I sometimes didn't get dressed at all and I didn't go out of the flat at all for days on end. I used to send the kids out to the shops. I stopped talking to the cat and I lost all interest in sex. It had always been very good between Barry and I but I just wasn't interested.

124

Then I read an article in the paper about people who were taking the Valium tablets and I remembered the name because that was what was on the bottle I'd been given. And they said that they were no better off than they were before they started them. Some said the pills were addictive like drugs. Several had the same symptoms as I had. They were all washed out and tired and not interested in anything.

I was so frightened by that that I just stopped taking the Valium there and then. I threw the pills down the toilet and put the bottle in the rubbish shute. I was frightened Barry would find out what I'd been taking and think I'd become a drug addict. I threw the newspaper article down the rubbish shute too. It was in our daily paper and I had to tell Barry that Tabby had been sick on it. Just sick on that page.

I thought I was going to die. I really did. I got this blinding headache and I couldn't stop shaking. I dropped Barry's chips all over the floor and he was ever so cross. I got dizzy too and was sick. It all happened quite quickly – within a few hours of my giving up the tablets.

It got worse all that evening and I didn't get to sleep at all that night. I can still remember it now. It was awful. I just lay there sweating and terrified. I don't know what I was terrified of but I was. I couldn't get up because I thought I'd fall over I was so dizzy. I was thirsty but I didn't want to drink because I thought I'd be sick again.

When Barry got up the next morning he wanted me to ring for the doctor but I wouldn't let him. I told him I'd be all right. But I wasn't. It got even worse. I had to draw the curtains because I couldn't bear the light and I felt really achey all over. I just sat in a chair all day and cried. Except that I couldn't cry properly. I wanted to cry but I couldn't.

When Barry came home he took one look at me and went straight out and called the doctor. The doctor wasn't pleased when he came. He said it was just flu and that Barry shouldn't have called him at that time of the day. He said it could have waited until the next day and that I should have gone to the surgery anyway. He gave me some aspirin tablets and some penicillin.

It went on for seven days like that. And then very slowly it began to get a bit better. Several times Barry wanted to call the doctor again but I begged him not to. I didn't want him near me. Barry was very good really.

The funny thing was that after about two days I suddenly realised what was wrong with me. I suddenly had this craving for the tablets I'd been taking. You know how you are when you're pregnant and you just suddenly have to have cucumber or something silly like that? Well, I wanted some Valium. I really wanted it. And then I remembered that article and I knew that what I was having was a 'withdrawal reaction' as they'd called it. That was another reason why I didn't want Barry to call the doctor. I was frightened that he'd find out that I'd been addicted to the Valium and that he'd be cross with me.

It's been a month now since I stopped the Valium and I still get dizzy occasionally but by and large I feel much better than I did. I still get very bored in the flat and I still get lonely and fed up. But I've been talking to Barry about it and I think if I keep at him he might let me get a little part-time job soon. I told him we could use the money for a holiday and he seemed to like the idea of that.

Mr. L.S.

I'd read a lot about the recession, of course, and I knew that there were millions of people who were unemployed but somehow it all seemed to be a problem that faced other people rather than me. Still can't believe the way it happened really because it was like one of those apocryphal stories that you hear people telling in the pub.

My job was in the personnel department and among other things I had the responsibility for drafting all the letters sent out by the company. You know, letters to tell people about changes in the pension plan, or about holiday arrangements and things like that. Well, one day someone came in and told me to prepare a general 'redundancy letter', for about two thousand men. A sort of communal 'Dear John' note. It was one of the worst jobs I've ever had to do because I knew that what I was writing in the letter wasn't strictly true. I was supposed to say that the reason for the redundancies was low productivity but in fact I knew that the company just wanted to sell off a huge factory site and realise a capital gain. We'd been bought up by an international holding company nine or ten months before and they weren't really interested in anything except a quick profit.

Well, to cut a sorry story as short as possible I got up a few days later to find one of those letters on my doormat.

I got a small redunadancy payment, of course, but it wasn't very much and I'd been working in the personnel department long enough to know that men of my age don't get jobs easily these days.

The money problem was real enough, of course. I'd never earned a lot but we'd always had enough to live on and we'd never really been short. But somehow it wasn't just the money that worried me. I can't properly explain how I felt but somehow it just seemed as though I'd been rejected. I've heard that some people who have been made redundant start off feeling quite optimistic about the future – thinking of all the jobs they'll be able to do. Well I never really went through that stage; probably because as I say I'd been in the personnel office long enough to know the truth. I just felt depressed and unwanted right from the start. I really was suicidal for a while. I really felt that I'd let the family down. That was the worst of it I suppose. The feeling that I'd failed the family and that they might suffer as a result. I didn't mention that to anyone, of course.

Marje, my wife, was very worried about me. I wasn't eating, I was losing weight and I was getting a lot of headaches. She took me along to the doctor. Unfortunately, our doctor doesn't speak much English and although I've got nothing against coloured doctors in themselves you understand it was all a bit of a waste of time. I'm not a racist but I couldn't understand what he was saying to me and he couldn't understand what I was saying to him. I might as well have been a cat at the vets.

Anyway, in the end he gave me some little white tablets and said they'd help me cope for a few months. He said that I could just ring the surgery if I wanted more and he'd put a prescription out in the porch for me. I suppose he was doing the best he could.

I didn't like those tablets right from the start but I thought I owed it to the doctor to give them a try so I persevered with them. They made me feel rather odd right from the first day I took them. It was as though I was outside my body looking in and watching someone else living there. That probably sounds stupid but it's how I felt.

They didn't make me sleepy and they didn't have any other effects at all. I carried on driving, I carried on doing everything just as normal. But I wasn't living my life any more. In a funny sort of way I suppose it helped me get over some of the worst of the depression because it distanced me from the real world. But the pills didn't solve anything and they didn't really help in the long term.

After I'd taken them for about ten days I decided that they weren't the answer so I stopped them. I thought about ringing up the doctor or going back but I decided against it in the end. I decided that I had to sort my problem out for myself so I bought an extendable ladder, a plastic bucket, a couple of wash cloths and a book of receipts and I started a window-cleaning business.

I put the ladder on the car roof, parked at the top of a different road each day and just worked my way up and down it. I felt a bit self-conscious at first because I'd always worked in an office and I'd always had what they call a white collar job but after a week I was enjoying myself. I was meeting people and I was my own boss. I earned quite a good bit that first week and I didn't have to work if the weather was bad because I had no boss to tell me what to do.

I still want something better but I've got my self-respect back now and at least I don't feel guilty about not bringing in a steady income. Some weeks I earn more than I did when I had a proper job! I quite realise that my solution might not suit everyone but for me it was a lot better than pills.

Mrs P.D.

When we got married I told my husband that I wanted to carry on with my career for a few years and he agreed that it would be a good idea. We both wanted a home of our own and we both wanted to have some money in the bank before we took on the responsibility of having children. I also wanted to have a career that I could go back to later on in my life. I didn't want to grow old and boring like so many women I know whose children have grown up.

Looking back I don't think my husband really understood how strongly I felt about my career for about six months after we'd got married he suggested that I stop taking the pill. He said he thought it was about time we started a family. Actually, I rather suspect that it was his mother who'd suggested the idea.

I reminded him that I had always intended to continue with my career for some time before getting pregnant and I explained that I was at a fairly critical point as far as my career was concerned. The competition in advertising is pretty tough and I'd just taken over a couple of fairly important accounts. I wanted a chance to show that I could handle them successfully.

Outwardly things went well enough after that but I honestly think that that was when our problems really started. I don't think my husband had understood just how determined I was to continue at the agency. He really seemed to hate my job. Looking back I suspect that he was a bit jealous too. I was earning quite a lot more than him and there weren't many opportunities for him at the Electricity Board. He'd done fairly well but was stuck in a bit of a middle management rut.

Well, all the obvious things happened then. I got fed up with the cold atmosphere at home so I started spending more and more time at the office and my husband got tired of waiting for me to come home and he started going to the local pub. Sometimes it would almost be as though we were having a competition to see who could get home latest. Before our marriage was a year old I was having an affair with one of the art directors at the agency and my husband was seeing a little too much of the barmaid at the local pub.

The divorce was as painless as things can be, I suppose. We just sold the house and all the furniture and divided the proceeds straight down the middle. Fortunately there were no children to worry about. Although I suppose you could say that if there had been we wouldn't have split up anyway.

It wasn't until about three months after the divorce had finally gone through that I started to feel bad about things. Looking back, I'm still not sure now whether or not I ever actually loved my husband but I think that I perhaps didn't give the marriage a fair chance.

Most of my friends told me that I was right to insist on carrying on my career. I had, after all, told my husband that I didn't want any children straight away. But deep down inside I wondered

129

whether I shouldn't have let him have a child early on. I really got quite depressed and upset about it for a while.

A skin rash I hadn't had since I'd been a girl came back and spread all over my hands and arms. It looked terrible. When I went to see my doctor and showed him the rash he asked if I'd had anything on my mind. I told him all about my problems at home and about the divorce and everything and he gave me some tablets to take. He said they wouldn't have any side effects or be addictive so I took them although I confess I was rather nervous about them. In fact, I remember that I went to the library and looked up the tablets in one or two textbooks. I even found some printed information that had been distributed by the manfuacturers. Everything that I read said that the pills were quite safe and that they weren't likely to cause any problems at all.

Well, they certainly helped get rid of my rash. But they took quite a bit of getting used to. When I first started to take them they made me feel quite odd and I needed to take half the dose the doctor had prescribed. If I took the full dose I just went to sleep all day. After about ten days, however, I managed to take the proper dose without too many problems.

Looking back I really don't know why I took the tablets at all. I knew why I'd got the skin rash – it was there because I'd been under a lot of stress. And I knew that there wasn't any way that a pill could help solve my problems. In fact I didn't really have any problem to be solved. I just had to come to terms with the fact that I'd had a disastrous marriage and needed time to get over it. But I suppose like everyone I liked the idea of a quick solution and my doctor had said that they'd be safe.

I took them for about three months in all and they changed my whole personality. I became careless about my work, I started to go out of the office and leave jobs half finished and I forgot appointments altogether sometimes. It all got so bad that Maurice, the art director I was going out with, suggested that I ought to see someone. He said he thought that I was suffering from depression or something as a result of the break-up of my marriage.

Well, I couldn't understand that at all. I honestly thought I'd got over the marriage. Everything really had gone quite amicably and there wasn't any of the nastiness that seems to characterise so many divorces these days. I knew I wasn't behaving rationally or normally but I didn't know why. I was actually getting quite unreasonably aggressive about little things. If my secretary didn't bring my coffee in just when I was expecting it I'd scream at her. It wasn't like me at all.

Then I went to a conference organised by a computer company I was doing some work for and while I was there I met a friend I hadn't seen for years. She saw me taking one of my tablets during a coffee break one morning and she went mad at me. She told me that I was really stupid to take the wretched things, wanted to know why I'd started them, how long I'd been taking them and everything.

That was the first I'd heard about them being really addictive and at first I didn't believe her. I told her that I'd looked them up and that my doctor had said that they were quite safe but she said that was all nonsense and that doctors and the drug companies were hand in hand. I thought that was a bit much but she was very convincing so I tried cutting down the pills as she suggested.

I think I must have cut them down a bit too quickly to start with because for forty-eight hours, I was really ill. I had the most awful shakes and it was a bit like a really bad hangover. I couldn't hold a pen and I couldn't put my lipstick on. My friend was very good and she said that I might as well go through it quickly rather than slowly but in retrospect I think it would have been wiser to take things a little more slowly. Anyway, she moved into my hotel room and stayed with me through the worst of it.

I honestly can't remember all that much about the conference and I can't remember how quickly or slowly I cut down the pills but I know it lasted for five or six days and when I came away I wasn't taking any pills at all. I felt really nervous when I left that place. If a dog barked within five hundred yards of me I jumped a mile. If anyone shouted or laughed I nearly jumped out of my skin. It was very eerie.

That feeling lasted for about a month or maybe a bit longer and then slowly it began to wear off. Then I started to feel slightly depressed about my broken marriage again. It was as though it had been there all the time and taking the tablets had just slowed down the whole process and spread it over a longer period. The skin rash even came back for a week or two.

131

It's all slowly getting better now but I've learned one lesson: next time I have a crisis I'll sort it out without my doctor's help, thank you very much.

Mrs O.B.

There's always been a lot of heart disease in our family. My dad died of a heart attack when he was fifty-five and my mum died of heart failure last year. She was seventy-eight but to be perfectly honest she hadn't really been what you'd call well for some time. My brother gets heart trouble too and he's been under the doctor for years now. About eleven years I think it is, to be precise. My dad had three heart attacks before he died and he was stuck in his chair for the last ten years of his life. A cardiac cripple they called him.

I got my first chest pains about twenty-four months ago when I was visiting my sister June in Preston. She's not been what you'd call a well woman either. She had a hysterectomy about fifteen years ago and to be perfectly honest she's never been well since then. She had a lot of 'chests' when she was a small girl and the doctor always said that she'd always have problems with her health. I was helping her clear out some stuff that she'd got in her garage when my pains came on. It was mostly stuff that had come from Uncle Harry's when he died back in 1979. He died of cancer of the throat but he had heart trouble too. There were some bits and pieces of furniture and five tea chests full of old books and what you might call knicks and knacks and bric à brac. He'd been in the merchant navy for about thirty years and he'd picked up all sorts of bits and pieces on his travels. A lot of it you'd probably call rubbish but there was a lovely lamp made of Venetian glass that I've got in my bedroom now. It's got a crack on one side but you can't see it unless you get really close and I keep that side nearest to the wall so you can't see it anyway.

The pains came on while we were moving one of the chests and they were right across my chest and down my arm. The pains that is. I know what the symptoms of heart disease are like because of my Dad.

June rang her doctor and he came round straight away. He was only young and he didn't examine me properly. He said that what

I'd done was strain a muscle and he said all I needed was a little rest. He gave me some pain killers with aspirin in that I can't take anyway and told me to take them every four hours.

Well, as soon as I got back home I went to see our proper doctor and got him to examine me. He had my vest off and gave me a thorough examination and check over but he said he couldn't find anything wrong with my heart either. That was quite a mystery because I know what the symptoms are like and I'd had a pain in my chest all right. He gave me some yellow tablets to help me relax and stop worrying and said they'd sort me out. He said I could keep on with them to stop the pains coming back.

I'd have probably still been taking them now but last Christmas my nephew James came to visit us. He's a nurse at one of the big London hospitals and when he heard my story he said I oughtn't to be taking the tablets at all but that I ought to have had some proper tests at the hospital. He rang up the doctor and made an appointment to go and see him.

To cut a long story short I got an appointment the following week to go and see a heart specialist at the hospital. He gave me a really thorough going-over and tested me with one of the electrical things like they have on the television. One of those things with the screen where you can see your heart beating. He showed me that there was absolutely nothing wrong with mine and it was a tremendous relief. I really believed him because he had all the latest equipment there.

He said I could stop the tablets too because they weren't doing me any good. I was glad about that because to be honest they hadn't done a thing for me except make me constipated. On reflection, I think my doctor only gave me the pills to keep me quiet and stop me worrying. If James hadn't come to visit I'd probably still be taking them now.

INDEX